ADVANCES IN
MEDICAL SOCIOLOGY

Volume 3 • 1993

THE SOCIAL
AND BEHAVIORAL ASPECTS
OF AIDS

ADVANCES IN
MEDICAL SOCIOLOGY

THE SOCIAL
AND BEHAVIORAL ASPECTS
OF AIDS

Volume Editors: GARY L. ALBRECHT
School of Public Health
University of Illinois at Chicago

RICK S. ZIMMERMAN
Department of Sociology
University of Miami

Series Editor: GARY L. ALBRECHT
University of Illinois at Chicago

VOLUME 3 • 1993

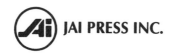 JAI PRESS INC.

Greenwich, Connecticut   *London, England*

CONTENTS

WHAT DOES AIDS TEACH US ABOUT SOCIAL SCIENCE?

Gary L. Albrecht and Rick S. Zimmerman

ABSTRACT

While many social problems share common characteristics, there are also considerable differences among them. This paper examines how behavioral science research on the social problem of AIDS can contribute to broader conceptual, theoretical, and methodological understandings of sociological phenomena. The study of AIDS reaffirms some fundamental principles of behavioral science but forces us to develop new approaches to examining health conditions. We situate the AIDS condition within the field of the sociology of health. We examine what AIDS is and means in different social, cultural, and political contexts. We discuss how AIDS raises many questions in the sociology of knowledge and development of science. We affirm that the study of AIDS produces research that has enormous policy implications and therefore raises fundamental questions concerning the interrelationships of science and policy. We explore how the study of AIDS forces us to re-evaluate our theories and models of behavior change. Finally, we indicate how AIDS may stimulate us to undertake research that will sharpen our theories, improve our methods, and lay the groundwork for informed social policy.

The Social and Behavioral Aspects of AIDS.
Advances in Medical Sociology, Volume 3, pages 1-18.
Copyright © 1993 by JAI Press Inc.
All Rights of reproduction in any form reserved.
ISBN: 1-55938-439-5

INTRODUCTION

When social scientists are confronted with a new phenomenon such as AIDS, they try to recast it in terms of existing paradigms and theories to make their work easier and familiar. New problems are often treated as interesting case studies of more fundamental processes. This intellectual approach has characterized much of the social science work on AIDS. Many assumptions were made and analyses undertaken with limited knowledge about or sensitivity to the peculiar phenomenon of AIDS.

AIDS has been defined as another social problem (Maris 1988; Hilgartner and Bosk 1988), analyzed for its social meaning (Conrad 1986), described in terms of lived experience (Weitz 1991; Siegel and Krauss 1991), seen as another stigmatizing condition (Lang 1990), used to study health education and models of behavior change (Fineberg 1988; Montgomery et al. 1989), and viewed as an epidemiological condition like Hepatitis B (Osborn 1989) or Tuberculosis (Goodgame 1990; Culotta 1991). Social scientists have used their accumulated knowledge and theoretical perspectives to inform the academic community and general public about AIDS. While such an approach is informative and in some cases helpful, it misses a major intellectual opportunity to see how the study of AIDS may push social scientists to modify familiar approaches to social problems and develop new theories and models.

Thus this paper does not focus on the topic of how social scientific theories and concepts in general, or within medical sociology in particular, can inform our understanding of HIV or of its social consequences. Rather, we examine how issues that have emerged as related to HIV and the study of HIV can inform our understanding of social science and the social scientific approach to health. Assisting the medical and public health communities in solving a variety of problems related to HIV (in the tradition of "sociology in medicine") has been and continues to be the priority for social scientists in general and for medical sociologists in particular. We believe, however, that it is now time to begin to step back and assess how behavioral science research on HIV can contribute to our broad conceptual, theoretical, and methodological perspectives and approaches to health in the behavioral sciences (in the tradition of "sociology of medicine").

AIDS AND THE SOCIOLOGY OF HEALTH

Social scientists use rhetoric and metaphors to convince the reader of the verisimilitude of their arguments (Atkinson 1990). In sociology this typically means that researchers present empirical findings in traditional formats to bolster their positions. The data presented are usually gathered through ethnographies in which the people are allowed to speak in their own words or through population based studies used to develop and test statistical models. In either case, the arguments are analogical and use a familiar rhetoric. Ethnographic studies rely on the power and credibility of informants to convince the reader. Population-based studies depend on the size and representativeness of the sample and power of the statistical model to draw strong inferences.

The metaphors used in the sociology of health typically define new conditions as another illness and disease. The argument is classically over who should control and define these conditions and whether or not they ought to be medicalized. When AIDS first came to the attention of the Centers For Disease Control and the press, it was seen as rare disease expressed through pneumonia and cancer in gay men. At this juncture AIDS was described as a gay disease represented by affluent young San Francisco and New York homosexual men. For men with HIV infection and the people in their lives AIDS, became a crisis. Thus, the popularization of the AIDS crisis metaphor. In the initial years of the condition, no one understood HIV infection well nor were there many useful protocols or effective drugs to treat AIDS. AIDS was seen as a death sentence to these gay men.

Soon, however, the picture became more complicated and people struggled for additional metaphors to characterize the condition. Many IV drug users in New York who shared needles began to appear as HIV positive, especially in the black and Hispanic communities. Shortly thereafter, their sexual partners began to manifest the condition. Given these data, most Americans, including sociologists, conceptualized AIDS as an epidemic of the gay and drug-using communities in large cities. Persons with AIDS were stigmatized with the mark of death. Infected persons were treated like lepers and avoided. The public took relief in the fact that AIDS was rampant only in the gay and drug using communities; that it was a condition of "deviants" and poor minorities and therefore was not of immediate concern to them. According to this metaphor, AIDS is a powerful sign because it embodied the multiple stigmas of sexual promiscuity, recreational drug-injecting, minority group membership in the black and Hispanic communities, and poverty. When the World Health Organization announced that 80 percent of AIDS cases worldwide were found in Africa and had been heterosexually transmitted, the Western public reacted in disbelief, did not attend to the facts because they concerned members of a remote, distinct population, or added Third World and African to the multiple stigma.

The recent history of AIDS has challenged the validity of these comfortable metaphors and called the rhetoric of science into question. Previously accepted assumptions of research, theory, and practice have been found wanting or oversimplifications of the reality. Medical sociologists can learn from the AIDS scientific enterprise. In fact, we can learn as much from studying the process and evolution of AIDS related research as we can facts about the condition itself.

The representation of a disease shapes research, policy, and public response (Gilman 1988). Characterizing AIDS as a gay and drug users' disease implicitly focused research and intervention programs on these populations while disregarding the vast majority of HIV positive people who have contracted the condition through unprotected heterosexual activity. Even as these facts become apparent, people talk about "safe sex," a metaphor meant to comfort, not to describe risk accurately. In the AIDS era, there is no such activity as safe sex unless one means total abstinence. Sex with a condom only reduces the risk. Condoms are often used incorrectly; they break, leak, and in some instances are permeable. Furthermore, sexually active individuals rarely report that they have used a condom every time they had sex over the last five years (Albrecht, Wells, and Valleron 1991). As cases of heterosexually transmitted HIV infection rapidly increase in the United States, we discover that scientists, practitioners, and the public have been lured by their metaphors to avoid confronting the hidden time bomb. Magic Johnson's candid announcement that he was HIV positive and contracted the condition through promiscuous heterosexual sex was deeply disconcerting because it notified everyone that their assumptions about AIDS were erroneous and their metaphors mechanisms to instill a false sense of security. As late as 1989, an internationally prominent epidemiologist declared that AIDS was not a major health problem because it was not highly infectious and was confined to the gay and drug-using communities. He said that these groups will suffer severe losses and the condition will have run its course; not to worry. The assumption was that the heterosexually active did not have to be concerned.[1] The metaphors and rhetoric on which he based his argument were appealing to many but faulty. Other conceptual models of illness were equally wanting in the case of AIDS. In epidemiology, medicine, and the social sciences, diseases are classically divided into infectious and chronic diseases; into mental and physical illnesses. AIDS was approached in this fashion but raised questions about this entire approach to the study of illness. AIDS is both an infectious and chronic disease. HIV infection jeopardizes the immune system resulting in a variety of opportunistic infections affecting physical health. Simultaneously, it affects the brain and causes symptoms that compromise psychological functioning.

From the beginning, AIDS was conceived as a condition that was contracted by individuals who were responsible for their behavior. But this is not always the case. Experience with the phenomenon shows that AIDS is a social disease. Individuals get AIDS by engaging in unprotected sexual intercourse, sharing needles with others when injecting recreational drugs, being born to an infected mother, and providing health care services to or receiving care from an infected individual. AIDS is contracted through social activities in which all parties often are not aware of the risk behaviors or HIV status of others. The unit of analysis for treatment and research ought to be dyads and interacting groups not isolated individuals. Until recently, few studies or programs target sexually active couples and needle-sharing networks. In this context, what does responsibility mean for the person high on drugs or alcohol, the monogamous wife who thinks that her husband is sexually faithful to her, the physician who does not know that her surgical patient is HIV infected, or to the baby born to the infected mother? These persons may not have recognized that they were even at risk when they engaged in an activity nor had control over the transmission event. On the other hand, there are instances of individuals who purposefully attempt to infect others out of spite or anger.

Most illness models operate on the assumption that if a person is ill, scientific medicine can diagnose the condition. The public is accustomed to believing that if they test negative for a condition, they do not have it. This is not true in the case of AIDS. There is considerable time between the time of first contact and seroconversion to HIV positive and from the point of seroconversion to manifestations of full-blown AIDS. Indeed, an estimated one million Americans are thought to be HIV positive and do not know it because they have not been tested and do not yet present AIDS symptoms. These facts have major consequences for research design and intervention programs (Albrecht 1989). Longitudinal population prospective study designs are required to follow the progression and conversion rate of the condition. In terms of intervention and treatment, testing negative now does not mean that the individual does not have the condition. Furthermore, just because persons have not contracted the condition does not mean that they will not if they persist in their risky behavior. Today's prevention will not make up for yesterday's indiscretions but it can protect others and prevent infection in the future.

Another common assumption is that AIDS is an illness that the medical community should control and treat. The fact is that medical professionals cannot control individual or group risk taking behavior, do not have an effective vaccine, are just beginning to understand the condition, and have but a few drugs and treatments that ameliorate symptoms and prolong life for those with the fatal condition. AIDS control will occur only when individuals change their risk behaviors and stop looking to medical science to solve the problem. AIDS is an clear example of a health problem where behavioral scientists have more to contribute to the control of the condition in the early stages than medical scientists. Indeed, the gay community of San Francisco organizing on a grass roots level probably did more to control HIV infection in their community than any scientists.

In spite of denial on the individual level, AIDS has received an amount of funding for research and treatment disproportionately larger than its incidence and prevalence would warrant. While AIDS is a major public health problem, the major causes of morbidity and mortality in the United States are heart disease, cancer, stroke, and suicide and homicide among young males. Breast cancer among women, smoking cessation, and control of firearms do not receive the funding or publicity of AIDS. The metaphors used to portray AIDS have captured attention and money disproportionate to the problem.

Within the sociology of health, AIDS has taught us that rhetoric and metaphors are important in science. But those metaphors developed on other social problems or medical conditions ought not to be applied to new problems without careful thought and exploratory work. AIDS has reminded us of the importance of choosing the most appropriate unit of analysis. AIDS research cautions us to avoid simple dichotomies in studying complex social and medical phenomena. The study of AIDS indicates that time and processes are variables often neglected in research. The San Francisco gay community underlined the power of grass roots movements in changing behavior and initiating a social movement. The brief history of AIDS demonstrates that the marketing of social problems has more effect on gathering attention and funding than morbidity and mortality statistics. Finally, experience with AIDS research suggests that we continually look for counterintuitive approaches to solve problems.

AIDS AND POLITICS

The brief history of AIDS underscores how deeply embedded politics are in research. The stakes in the AIDS business are huge. On the biological level, there are Nobel prizes to be won for those that can unravel the immunological puzzles presented by the HIV virus. For social scientists, careers can be made by developing behavior-change and intervention models that will result in reducing risk behaviors in the population. Within universities, the millions of dollars of indirect cost recovery from funded research translates into fiscal health for schools experiencing hard economic times and raises, promotions, and tenure for the principal investigators who attracted the money. Governments have the reputation of their national laboratories at stake. In the case of AIDS, the federal government and pharmaceutical companies also generate hundreds of millions of dollars from HIV tests and AIDS-related drugs that were "discovered" in government research institutes and subsequently patented. The struggle for control over the AIDS business is even felt on the international level. The top management of the Global Programme On AIDS at the World Health Organization in Geneva was drastically reorganized in March 1990 in a dispute over who was to control the effort and program priorities. Observers are not convinced that this bureaucratic upheaval was even constructive (Placa 1991a).

The infusion of politics into science is also exemplified by the Gallo controversy at the National Institutes of Health. A competitive race between the Montangier team at the Pasteur Institute in Paris and the Gallo team at the U.S. National Institutes of Health to identify the HIV virus and develop diagnostic tests for it resulted in a major scientific scandal. In the early 1980s, both teams were thought to have discovered the HIV virus at about the same time. Both teams were credited with the work and the French and U.S. governments shared profits from the patents based on this work. Recently, however, serious allegations of scientific misconduct were raised when it became public that the Gallo virus seems to have been "misappropriated" from the Pasteur labs and used in the development and manufacture of the HIV blood test later patented by the U.S. government. After a two-year investigation, the NIH is preparing to close the case without having satisfactorily examined the central question: "Did someone in the Gallo laboratory steal the HIV virus discovered by the Pasteur team?" (Crewdson 1991). The investigation did uncover that critical data seem to have been falsified or fabricated in the NIH labs and that investigators may not have even carefully read the papers on which their names appeared before they were published. By any standard, politics and competition seem to have compromised science.

AIDS also demonstrates that the choice of research topics can elicit volcanic political reactions from the political bodies that fund such work. In 1990 and 1991, conservatives in Congress led by Jesse Helms stymied two studies important for understanding how to intervene in reducing AIDS risk behaviors among adolescents and how to change people's risky sexual behavior. Both the University of North Carolina study to examine adolescent sexual behavior and the National Opinion Research Center (NORC) study to identify adult sexual behavior passed scientific peer review but were not funded because they were thought by some members of Congress and the White House to ask questions that were offensive and too sensitive. As a consequence, the Surgeon General and public-health officials must base their AIDS intervention efforts and policies on skimpy and incomplete data. In this case, sexual politics won over scientific merit.

So much for value-free science. Research has become a big business with substantial rewards to the winners. Traditional academic and scientific values have taken a buffeting. Prizes, favored positions, and money go to those in power, those who control and direct the research efforts. Since the competition is intense, research entrepreneurs are driven by "move it or lose it" values just like other business persons (Toffler 1991). The "move it or lose it" values are espoused by managers in highly competitive market niches that must get results immediately or risk losing their group market position or even their jobs. They impart the message to subordinates, "Get the job done on time and I will not ask questions about how you did it." What can we learn from the history of AIDS science? Any remaining illusions that science is value free have been publicly shattered. Political ideologies of those that control funding and government programs define the problem and the types of research done. Attention is focused away from the facts toward interpretations of the facts. While power struggles rage over who will control and profit from the AIDS business, those with the disease struggle along having to fight widespread discrimination and are often forced to help themselves or be abandoned.

SOCIOLOGY OF SCIENCE/KNOWLEDGE

One classic problem in the sociology of science is the possibility that by merely measuring or observing an object, the object is necessarily affected, yielding results that no longer truly reflect the object before it was observed. In the physical sciences, it has been termed the Heisenberg principle; in the behavioral sciences, examples have been described as the "Hawthorne effect," demand effects, interviewer effects, and methods effects. There are at least two ways that scientific research on HIV may itself have an impact on HIV-related awareness and/or behavior. First, conducting interviews may have an influence on people's perceptions. By raising issues of attitudes, beliefs, or knowledge, the researcher may be bringing into awareness issues not yet considered or previously left unresolved by the respondent. Second, mass media reports of scientific research about HIV may indirectly have effects on HIV-related attitudes, knowledge, and behavior. Much research has focused on intended effects of the mass media on increased awareness and understanding of HIV (Flora and Maibach 1990; Wellings 1988; Stipp and Kerr 1989; Kinsella 1990; Baker 1986). To the extent that the mass media have been increasingly reporting work on vaccines and/or cures, this reporting may have a negative impact on people's behavior. Recent evidence from the National Center for Health Statistics suggests that reports during the last year about progress on cures and vaccines may have increased misperceptions about the current availability of a vaccine. The proportion who did not know that it was definitely false that there is a vaccine for the AIDS virus increased from 25 percent in late 1989 to nearly one-third in mid-1990 (Adams and Hardy 1991). Because beliefs about cures and vaccines have been shown to be related to behavioral attitudes and behaviors (Becker and Joseph 1988), media reports may have indirectly had a negative consequence on HIV-related risk behavior. This research also shows that the proportion of individuals who say they have received information about AIDS/HIV from mass media sources (television, radio, magazines, and newspapers) has decreased 5 to 10 percent between March and September 1990, with an increase from 9 to 13 percent saying they have received no information on AIDS in the past month. Thus, ongoing changes in patterns of mass media reports about AIDS/HIV, as well as unintended consequences, appear to be occurring at present.

Yet another way in which the evolution of research on AIDS may contribute to our understanding of the scientific process, and may indeed change it, is through consumers' involvement in research. Perhaps as never before, those affected by the disease have lobbied to have input into the ethical and economic issues concerning research on HIV with human subjects. FDA rules concerning the development of new drugs have been modified dramatically to enable those with a terminal illness (including, at present, AIDS) to gain access to experimental drugs more quickly in their development than ever before. Concerns about the exclusion of women and the underrepresentation of minorities in drug trials have led to new regulations concerning the recruitment of participants for clinical trials.

BEHAVIORAL SCIENCE RESEARCH, AIDS, AND PUBLIC POLICY

In an ideal world, behavioral science research would discover the important correlates of risky behavior, the groups of individuals in whom that behavior was occurring, the environment and situational contexts in which it is most difficult to modify, and suggest means of changing the behavior. Instead, various groups sometimes use research results to "lie with statistics" and "political correctness" defines what hypotheses are appropriate to be tested, what results are appropriate to be reported, and from what perspective they should be reported. The questions of rates of HIV seropositivity among Haitian-Americans, homosexual versus heterosexual men, those who reside in the ghettos versus in the suburbs, and those who are prostitutes or IV drug users versus those who are not are not politically correct questions in 1991, and they are not likely to be politically correct questions any time soon. The distinction between "risk behaviors" and "risk groups" was delineated very early on in the epidemic so that certain groups would not be stigmatized and that others outside of those groups would not feel their risk to be zero. The conclusion to be drawn from this distinction was that every citizen of the United States and, in fact, the world, is at risk, and since anyone could engage in risk behaviors, the message needs to be communicated to all. This same logic would have us direct stop smoking campaigns at the general public though we know that minority members are not quitting as often as whites and especially that young women have been starting to smoke in alarming numbers. As described by Fumento (1990) in his *The Myth of Heterosexual AIDS,* the spread of HIV throughout the heterosexual community has generally been over-dramatized in a number of ways, probably in order to maximize concern about AIDS in general. The political realities have superseded the public health reality in the use of behavioral-science research results to develop public policy. Of course, as representatives of the public health community, we should prudently add that as the majority of cases of AIDS in the world were contracted through heterosexual sex and since we do not know the true incidence of HIV in the heterosexual community, the heterosexual, sexually active general public should still be cautious about their behaviors.

Another problematic issue concerning behavioral science research and public policy concerns effective intervention. By virtue of a strong and early commitment to behavioral science research, including an evaluation component, the gay community was able to document the "effectiveness" of its behavioral-oriented approach to behavior change. Dramatic changes in attitudes with concurrent and equally dramatic changes in behavior—for example, greater condom use and fewer partners (cf. Becker and Joseph 1988)—were shown relatively early. As a result, despite the fact that a majority of new diagnosed cases of AIDS were among homosexual and bisexual men, funding agencies were moving on to other groups, including women and minorities. Yet, recent research (Kelly, St. Laurence, and Brasfield 1991) suggests that "relapse," that is, return to consistently unsafe sexual behavior or occasional unsafe sexual behavior, is relatively common among gay men, as indeed it is among most groups affected by risk-related behavior change, and therefore warrants continued attention.

HIV-RELATED BEHAVIOR CHANGE AND INTERVENTIONS

A further assumption is that existing behavior-change models apply well to AIDS. Most of these models are based on communications theory and cognitive psychology. Proponents of these models argue that if people are sensitized to the risk, have accurate knowledge, and manifest appropriate attitudes, they will change their high-risk behaviors. AIDS knowledge, attitudes, perceptions, and behavior research shows that this is not necessarily so. The situational context of the encounter, emotions, and denial affect these behaviors.

We have learned that rational models do not explain AIDS risk-taking behaviors well. Research on behavior change among gay men in San Francisco brought into focus the potential importance of peer norms, a variable from Fishbein and Ajzen's Theory of Reasoned Action (1975; Ajzen and Fishbein 1980) that has been around for at least two decades but was recently rediscovered by researchers more familiar with the Health-Belief Model. Similarly, emotions have been added into various models to explain HIV-related behavior; other researchers have argued for decades about the importance of emotion as it relates to risk reducing behavior (cf. Leventhal and Scherer 1987), but HIV has brought greater attention to this variable (Dworkin, Albrecht, and Cooksey 1991).

An empirically-based approach to model development has led to less theoretically narrow models. The AIDS Risk-Reduction Model is a good example (Catania, Kegeles, and Coates 1990). In the field of health promotion and prevention generally, the Health Belief Model was determined to be at a turning point almost ten years ago by its authors; yet, researchers go about attempting to test the model intact. Other models that do not focus on risk perception per se—such as Ajzen and Fishbein's model or social learning theory models—may contribute to a better understanding of HIV-related risk behavior, and in so doing may lead researchers in other areas of prevention (e.g., cancer, CHD, diabetes, mental illness) to discover variables beyond those within their discipline of training. At the same time, the discovery of a more empirically-based approach to model-building should lead to more behavior-specific models, or at least models developed for classes of behaviors. It has always seemed a bit odd to think that the processes that lead a person to engage in regular exercise would also lead a person to use a sunblock to reduce the risk of cancer or use less salt in their food. So, for example, if HIV-related behavior tends to involve other people, the model should include interpersonal and/or sociostructural variables. If the purchase of condoms or exercise equipment or clothes or sunblock requires a certain level of economic resources, then economic variables should be included in the pertinent behavior change model. To the extent that HIV-related behaviors are a bit different from those related to CHD or cancer, research on HIV-related behavior may lead researchers to discover that models designed for one set of behaviors may not be equally applicable to another set of behaviors.

AIDS has also reminded (or better, awakened) prevention researchers to the important realization that individual behavior change does not occur in a vacuum but rather in an interpersonal, cultural, and societal context. The papers by Kayal, Aggleton, and Friedman (this volume) discuss related issues. Perceptions of one's sex partner as well as one's sex partner's perceptions, the nature of the relationship with one's sex partners, and peer norms affect one's attitudes, intentions, and behaviors. Similarly, cultural context interacts with beliefs in producing behavior. The meaning of premarital sex, the act of sexual intercourse, a sexual relationship, the use of condoms or birth control devices, anal intercourse, and sharing needles for IV drug use may have significantly different meanings for individuals depending on their cultural heritage. As a result, successful interventions are increasingly taking cultural factors into account. Socioeconomic, political, and sociohistorical contexts are also important for understanding and predicting HIV-related behavior, as they are for understanding and predicting many kinds of health-related behavior. Given the strong historical, political, and economic influences on individuals' choices and behaviors related to HIV, research on HIV-related behavior change may force attention to these domains when research is conducted on prevention of other diseases.

THE CULTURAL RELATIVITY AND INSENSITIVITY OF AIDS INTERVENTIONS AND RESEARCH

AIDS also points out the limitations of culturally biased research. Most early social research on AIDS was conducted in the United States and Western Europe where the high-risk populations were gay men and IV drug users who shared needles for injecting. Science and intervention strategies were based on these studies and taken around the world. The problem is that over 70 percent of AIDS cases around the world resulted from heterosexual activity. The interventions designed for gay and drug-using populations were not equally applicable to the heterosexual populations that account for the majority of AIDS cases without serious modifications (Culotta 1991). The HIV-infection rate among Asian prostitutes is skyrocketing (McDermott 1991). Males in Zaire and Uganda do not perceive condoms to be central in combatting AIDS and they continue to have unprotected sex with multiple female partners (Bertrand et al. 1991; Perlez 1991). Throughout Africa, as young people migrate from rural areas to cities, they increase their unprotected promiscuous sexual activity even though they know the risk for AIDS (Careal, Cleland, Denheneffe, and Adeokun 1990). Health education programs developed in Western nations have not been effective in changing behaviors in these populations.

Critics state that the major interest of Western scientists in Africa is in doing "safari" research, studies that cannot be done for ethical or economic reasons in developed countries (Placa 1991b). "Helicopter researchers" drop in an African village, collect data, and exit without leaving anything behind to ameliorate the inherent AIDS problem. Such work is not sensitive to the needs of persons with AIDS or individuals in different cultures. For instance, how does a Western researcher get informed consent from illiterate respondents? Proposed vaccine trials reinforce accusations of cultural insensitivity. The countries preliminarily selected for these international trials are Rwanda, Uganda, Zaire, Thailand, and Brazil (Cohen 1991).

METHODOLOGICAL ISSUES

Because research on HIV concerns private behaviors that are generally considered socially undesirable by society and, at least early on, involved groups for which a sampling frame does not exist, research on AIDS has led researchers to attempt to tackle some thorny methodological questions (Catania, Gibson, Chitwood, and Coates 1990). A classic methodologic question and one still not very clearly answered in sociology concerns how best to ask questions about sensitive topics. Recent handbooks of survey methodology (Frey 1983; Backstrom and Hursh-Cesar 1981) suggest that the self-administered questionnaire may be more effective in eliciting valid responses than face-to-face interviews because of possible concern in interviews that anonymity may be compromised. Other research suggests that interviews may yield more reporting of socially undesirable behavior because of the development of rapport and trust between the respondent and the researcher via the interviewer. In a recent, unpublished study, Cabral, Zimmerman, and Langer found that respondents in an STD clinic were more likely to report using crack or paying for sex with money or drugs when they were interviewed than when they filled out an anonymous self-administered questionnaire. Further research should probably assess and/or experimentally manipulate the conditions and contexts in which each survey method may yield more valid results.

Because reports concerning HIV-related risk behaviors may have life and death consequences, other methods of improving validity of self-reports have also been used. The random response technique is an elaborate method which has been found to improve the reporting rate concerning sensitive behaviors or socially undesirable attitudes (Tracy and Fox 1981). Very briefly, it is a technique that allows respondents to give answers that they know make it impossible for the researcher to link the sensitive or socially undesirable behavior or attitude to them. It allows for the estimation of rates within a population, but does not permit individual-level modeling of data. Thus, this method could be used to estimate prevalence of sexual behavior and to allow for comparisons between subgroups. A variation of the random response technique, called the "item/count paired lists technique," developed by Miller (1984; Miller and Cisin 1984) is less cumbersome and has been used to estimate the prevalence of drug use. In this approach the respondent is given a list of behaviors, which includes the sensitive behavior of interest and a host of innocuous items, and is instructed to report the total number of activities in the list he or she has participated in. A second, randomly selected sample of respondents is given a similar list, but with the sensitive trait removed. Consequently, by subtracting the mean counts between the two samples, an estimate of the prevalence of the sensitive behavior is obtained. This technique has been found by the second author (Zimmerman and Langer 1992) to increase by 50 percent (from 9% to almost 14%) the estimated prevalence of sexual behavior with a member of the same sex. The importance of valid reports as they relate to HIV has led researchers to develop and/or apply validity-increasing methods which are likely to be useful in other contexts.

As qualitative research has begun to be fashionable again in medical sociology (Mechanic 1990), such studies on AIDS have burgeoned. Research on substantive topics such as "deviant subcultures and careers" and coping with chronic illness has traditionally used qualitative methods; since AIDS involves both of these elements, it naturally has been amenable to qualitative study. The papers by Broadhead and Fox and by Weitz in (this volume) are good examples of the rich description and understanding made possible by qualitative research—whether participant observation, diaries, ethnography, or semi-structured interviewing.

Given the necessity for some AIDS research (such as that involving gay men or IV drug users) to construct "representative" samples of hidden or difficult-to-find populations, a variety of sampling strategies have been developed or used that are likely to benefit other research in the behavioral sciences. At least two such methods have been used in AIDS research: snowball sampling within a probability sampling frame and screening for rare populations. Snowball sampling has been around for a long time. This is a sampling technique where the researcher discovers a small number of informants to interview, then has those informants lead him/her to other informants, and so on (except for Miami students and others who have never seen snow, the "snowball" metaphor applies rather well, with each successive generation of informants larger than the last). Martin and Dean (1985) used the snowball sampling procedure more carefully than others have done so, documenting the characteristics of each successive snowball generation. They began by enumerating gay-associated organizations in the New York area; they constructed a stratified sample of organizations and had those organizations construct a systematic, random sample of their members, sending questionnaires to the sampled members. Then, those individuals were asked to solicit three of their friends not in that organization to complete questionnaires, and so on. Five or more successive snowball generations were constructed; it turned out that each was less centrally located in the network of individuals in the sample, improving upon the earlier informants as a representative group. Probability and nonprobability methods were combined, and a nonprobability method was as carefully documented and described as it has ever been. These techniques developed for AIDS research are applicable to other topics as well.

Screening for a rare population (Sudman 1976, pp. 200-210) has been previously identified as a technique used to yield completed interviews with members of a subpopulation that comprises only a small proportion of those in the overall population. Using this method, the researcher conducts a brief screening interview at the beginning of the interview (generally a phone interview); those respondents who are members of the intended population then receive the remainder of the phone interview while for those who are not members of the group of interest, the interview is ended. Montgomery, Lewis, and Kirchgraber (1991) used this method successfully, as has the Research and Decisions Corporation, in identifying gay males for phone interviews.

Another lesson we can learn from research on HIV prevention is that relationships found between variables cross-sectionally may not appear longitudinally. Research by Joseph and colleagues (Emmons et al. 1986) showed strong relationships cross-sectionally between knowledge and a variety of attitudes on the one hand and HIV risk behavior on the other. Longitudinal analyses of Multicenter AIDS Cohort Study (MACS) data (Joseph et al. 1987), however, found weaker and far fewer significant relationships than those based on cross-sectional data. Retrospective reporting was discovered to have lead to inflated correlations.

A related and fairly technical, but potentially important, development is the creation of reliable, unique subject identifiers for anonymous but longitudinal research (which thus requires the linking of questionnaires over time). This involves the use of information that subjects are unlikely to believe can be traced and linked to their name but which subjects will consistently report over time. Variables such as mother's maiden name, number of older brothers and sisters, and day (but not month) of birth have been used successfully. This method can be used for other research topics where potential sensitiveness of the information would be a respondent concern but where linking of data over time is important.

WHAT HAVE WE LEARNED?

The study of AIDS has taught us that intellectual imperialism has its limitations. When assumptions, theories, and models that have been developed on problems in the United States are unilaterally applied to other social and cultural contexts, they are often found wanting or even naive. For new or more sophisticated models to be generated, more attention should be given to inductive research. Extensive first-hand, on-site observations over protracted periods of time are to establish basic descriptive information before theories and models can be constructed and large sample surveys profitably undertaken. Let the people speak and tell us what they experience before we try to interpret their behavior. New insights are more likely to arise out of the field in the study of AIDS than through armchair theorizing at this stage of the condition. Established rhetoric and metaphors do not substitute for a fresh view or a different perspective.

We have also learned that social problems are not isomorphic. Whenever we encounter a new social problem, we should be reluctant to apply "off the shelf" analytical tools from our intellectual workshop. While many social problems share common characteristics, there are also considerable differences among them. AIDS illustrates that more attention can also be fruitfully given to groups of social problems that cluster together. Experience with AIDS research continually reminds us that existing theories of behavior change, the effect of emotions on behavior, perceptions of invulnerability, ambiguity, stigma, attribution of responsibility, and stratification of disease in society need reconsideration.

Politics and unbridled competition can destroy science. Researchers lose credibility when their pursuit of rewards and prominence supplants their pursuit of truth. The public fight over findings, patents, and profits in the AIDS business suggests to the public that self-interest is more important than the advancement of science or assistance of those with a lethal condition. AIDS also brings questions of ethics and values to the forefront. Some of the questions raised are: Do the same rules of research apply in Third World countries as at home? Of what value is a human life? How much medical care is reasonable in a given situation? Who is responsible for AIDS? Do health care workers have an obligation to treat AIDS patients and should society pay for this care? For the academic and research communities, AIDS questions whether or not truth and validity are more important than getting there first, receiving the prize, or controlling the field. The race to succeed has forced us to ask whom and what we can believe.

Finally, AIDS research makes some of the historical debate about sociology in medicine and sociology of medicine seem dated. AIDS is simultaneously a medical and social condition. Without high-technology medicine and immunological research, we would not know the pathophysiology of HIV infection. But at present, medicine is helpless in preventing the spread of the disease. In fact, behavioral scientists have more to offer the intervention and prevention of AIDS than does medicine. This situation has forced interdisciplinary research. AIDS is larger than the study of medicine or health; it involves fundamental questions concerning sex, drugs, poverty, stigma, discrimination, responsibility for behavior, and allocation of resources in a stratified society.

NOTE

1. This remark was made in confidence so the source will remain anonymous.

REFERENCES

Adams, P.R. and A.M. Hardy. 1991. "AIDS Knowledge and Attitudes for July- September 1990." Provisional data from the NHIS. Advance data from vital and health statistics, No. 198. Hyattsville, MD: U.S. Public Health Service.
Ajzen, I. and M. Fishbein. 1980. *Understanding Attitudes and Predicting Social Behavior.* Englewood Cliffs, NJ: Prentice-Hall.
Albrecht, G.L. 1989. "The Intelligent Design of AIDS Research Strategies." Pp. 67-74 in *Health Services Research Methodology: A Focus On AIDS,* edited by L. Sechrest, H. Feeeman, and A. Mulley. Washington, DC: NCHSR.
Albrecht, G.L., J. Wells, and A.J. Valleron. 1991. "HIV Risk Behaviors Among Adolescents/ Adults In Three Countries: France, U.K., and U.S." Paper presented at the VII International AIDS Conference, Florence, Italy.
Atkinson, P. 1990. *The Ethnographic Imagination: Textual Construction of Reality.* London: Routledge.
Baker, A.B. 1986. "The Portrayal of AIDS in the Media: An Analysis of Articles in the New York Times. Pp. 179-194 in *The Social Dimension of AIDS: Method and Theory,* edited by D.A. Feldman and M. Johnson. New York: Praeger.

Becker, M.H. and J. Joseph. 1988. "AIDS and Behavioral Change to Reduce Risk: A Review." *American Journal of Public Health* 78: 394-410.

Backstrom, C.H., and G. Hursh-Cesar. 1981. *Survey Research* (2nd ed.). New York: John Wiley.

Bertrand, J.T., B. Makani., S.E. Hassig, K. Niwembo, B. Djunghu, M. Muanda, and C. Chirhamolekwa. 1991. "AIDS-Related Knowledge, Sexual Behavior, and Condom Use Among Men and Women In Kinshasa, Zaire." *American Journal of Public Health* 81: 53-58.

Careal, M., J. Cleland, J.C. Denheneffe, and L. Adeokun. November 1990. "Research On Sexual Behavior That Transmits HIV: The GPA/WHO Collaborative Surveys." Paper presented at the World Health Organization Seminar, Sonderborg, Denmark.

Catania, J., D.R. Gibson, D.D. Chitwood, and T.J. Coates. 1990. "Methodological Problems in AIDS Behavioral Research: Influences on Measurement Error and Participation Bias in Studies of Sexual Behavior." *Psychological Bulletin* 108: 339-362.

Catania, J., S. Kegeles, and T. Coates. 1990. "Towards an Understanding of Risk Behavior: An AIDS Risk Reduction Model (AARM)." *Health Education Quarterly* 17: 381-399.

Cohen, J. 1991. "AIDS Vaccine Meeting: International Trials Soon." *Science* 254: 647.

Conrad, P. 1986. "The Social Meaning of AIDS." *Social Policy* 14: 51-56.

Crewdson, J. 1991. "AIDS Probe Nears End: Key Question Remains." *Chicago Tribune* (November 17), pp. 1, 20.

Culotta, E. 1991. "Forecasting the Global AIDS Epidemic." *Science* 253: 852-854.

Dworkin, J., G. Albrecht, and J. Cooksey. 1991. "Concern about AIDS among Hospital Physicians, Nurses and Social Workers." *Social Science and Medicine* 33: 239-248.

Emmons, C., J. Joseph, R. Kessler, C. Wertman, S. Montgomery, and D. Ostrow. 1986. "Psychosocial Predictors of Reported Behavior Change in Homosexual Men at Risk for AIDS." *Health Education Quarterly* 13: 331-345.

Fineberg, H.V. 1991. "Education To Prevent AIDS: Prospects and Obstacles." *Science* 239: 592-596.

Fishbein, M. and I. Ajzen. 1975. *Belief, Attitude, Intention, and Behavior: An Introduction to Theory and Research*. Reading, MA: Addison-Wesley.

Flora, J.A. and E.W. Maibach. 1990. "Cognitive Responses to AIDS Information: The Effects of Issue Involvement and Message Appeal." *Communication Research* 17: 759-774.

Frey, J.H. 1983. *Survey Research by Telephone*. Beverly Hills, CA: Sage.

Fumento, M. 1990. *The Myth of Heterosexual AIDS: How a Tragedy has been Distorted by the Media and Partisan Politics*. New York: Basic Books.

Gilman, S.L. 1988. *Disease and Representation: Images of Illness From Madness to AIDS*. Ithaca, NY: Cornell University Press.

Goodgame, R.W. 1990. "Aids In Uganda-Clinical and Social Features." *New England Journal of Medicine* 323: 383-389.

Hilgartner, S. and C.L. Bosk. 1988. "The Rise and Fall of Social Problems: A Public Arenas Model." *American Journal of Sociology* 94: 53- 8.

Joseph, J., S. Montgomery, C. Emmons, R. Kessler, D. Ostrow, C. Wortman, M. O'Brien, and S. Ishleman. 1987. "Magnitude and Determinants of Behavioral Risk Reduction: Longitudinal Analysis of a Cohort at Risk for AIDS." *Psychology and Health* 1: 73-96.

Kelly, J.A., J.S. St. Laurence, and T.L. Brasfield, T.L. 1991. "Predictors of Vulnerability to AIDS Risk Behavior Relapse." *Journal of Consulting and Clinical Psychology* 59: 163-166.

Kinsella, J. 1990. *Covering the Plague: AIDS and the American Media*. New Brunswick, NJ: Rutgers University Press.

Lang, N.G. 1990. "Sex, Politics, and Guilt: A Study of Homophobia and the AIDS Phenomenon." Pp. 169-182 in *Culture and AIDS*, edited by D.A. Feldman. Westport, CT: Greenwood Press.

Leventhal, H. and K. Scherer. 1987. "The Relationship of Emotion to Cognition: A Functional Approach to a Semantic Controversy." *Cognition and Emotion* 1: 3-28.

Maris, R.W. 1988. *Social Problems.* Chicago: The Dorsey Press.

Martin, J. and L. Dean. 1985. "The Impact of AIDS on Gay Men in New York City: The Development of a Community Sample." Paper presented at the American Public Health Association Conference, Washington, DC., November.

McDermott, J. 1991. "Asia—The Smoldering Volcano." *AIDS and Society* 2: 1,4.

Mechanic, D. 1989. "Medical Sociology: Some Tensions among Theory, Method, and Substance." *Journal of Health and Social Behavior* 30: 147-160.

Miller, J.P. 1981. "Complexities of the Randomized Response Solution." *American Sociological Review* 46: 928-930

Miller, J.D. and I.H. Cisin. 1984. "The Item-count/paired Lists Technique: An Indirect Method of Surveying Deviant Behavior." Unpublished manuscript, Social Research Group, George Washington University, Washington, DC.

Montgomery, K., C.E. Lewis, and P. Kirchgraber. 1991. "Telephone Screening for Risk of HIV Infection." *Medical Care* 29: 399-407.

Montgomery, S.B., J.G. Joseph, M.H. Becker, D.G. Ostrow, R.C. Kessler, and J.P. Kirscht. 1989. "The Health Belief Model in Understanding Compliance With Preventive Recommendations For AIDS: How Useful?" *AIDS Education and Prevention* 1: 303-323.

Osborn, J.E. 1989. "A Risk Assessment of the AIDS Epidemic." Pp. 23-38 in V.M. Mays, G.W. Albee, and S.F. Schneider (eds.), *Primary Prevention of AIDS.* Newbury Park, CA: Sage.

Perlez, J. 1990. "Toll of AIDS On Uganda's Women Puts Their Roles and Rights In Question." *New York Times International*(October 28).

Placa, J. 1991a. "WHO AIDS Program: Moving On a New Track." *Science* 254: 511-512.

_____. 1991b. "African AIDS: Whose Research Rules?" *Science* 250: 199-201.

Research and Decisions Corporation. 1985. *A Report on Designing an Effective AIDS Prevention Campaign Strategy for San Francisco: Results from the Second Probability Sample of an Urban Gay Male Community.* San Francisco, CA: Research and Decisions Corporation.

Siegel, K. and B.J. Krauss. 1991. "Living With the HIV Infection: Adaptive Tasks of Seropositive Gay Men." *Journal of Health and Social Behavior* 32: 17-32.

Stipp, H. and D. Kerr. 1989. "Determinants of Public Opinion about AIDS. *Public Opinion Quarterly* 53: 98-106.

Sudman, S. 1976. *Applied Sampling.* New York: Academic Press.

Toffler, B.L. 1991. "When The Signal Is 'Move It or Lose It.'" *The New York Times Forum* (November 17), p. 13.

Tracy, P.E. and J.A. Fox. 1981. "The Validity of Randomized Response for Sensitive Measurements." *American Sociological Review* 46: 187-200.

Weitz, R. 1991. *Life With AIDS.* New Brunswick, NJ: Rutgers University Press.

Wellings, K. 1988. "Perceptions of Risk: Media Treatment of AIDS." Pp. 83-107 in *Social Aspects of AIDS,* edited by P. Aggleton and H. Homans. London: The Falmer Press.

Zimmerman, R.S. and L.M. Langer. 1992. "Improving Prevalence Estimates of Sensitive Behaviors: The Randomized Lists Technique and Self-reported Honesty." Manuscript submitted for publication.

AIDS AS A SOCIOHISTORICAL
PHENOMENON

Samuel R. Friedman

ABSTRACT

Macrosociological, sociohistorical, and middle-range social forces have shaped
the course of the HIV epidemic—as evidenced by markedly different
sociodemographic patterns in the degree of AIDS case prevalence, HIV
seroprevalence, risk behaviors, and risk reduction. Nevertheless, individualistic
and microsocial models have so far been near-hegemonic in public-health policy
and programs. Moreover, despite evidence that collective self-organization has
been the key factor in the relative success of gay community responses to AIDS,
and that projects based on middle-range approaches have been unusually
successful in interventions with drug injectors, to date little has been done to
apply the lessons learned through these experiences more systematically or on
a wider scale. Historical, macrosociological, and middle-range research should
be pursued and applied in this epidemic, and the knowledge gained thereby may
stengthen our more general research enterprise. In addition, efforts must be made
to challenge the overly individualistic approaches taken by public-health agencies
and, indeed, by American behavioral research.

The Social and Behavioral Aspects of AIDS.
Advances in Medical Sociology, Volume 3, pages 19-36.
Copyright © 1993 by JAI Press Inc.
All Rights of reproduction in any form reserved.
ISBN: 1-55938-439-5

INTRODUCTION

Much of medical sociology tends to view the individual as an isolated monad, or at most encompasses the interaction of the individual with his or her most immediate social environment, even in its treatment of AIDS and other epidemics that plainly involve interpersonal transmission of disease-causing agents. This paper, however, will argue that larger-scale social structures have more to do with the fates and behaviors of individuals at risk for AIDS than do the microsocial variables that are emphasized by health beliefs models (Becker and Joseph 1988; Emmons et al. 1986; Montgomery et al. 1989) or by social learning theory (Bandura 1977; Botvin, Baker, Botvin, Filazzola, and Millman 1984; Des Jarlais and Friedman 1988; Evans 1976). Furthermore, there is a fundamentally historical component to this epidemic, and historical contexts are likely to be crucial in shaping other instances of widespread morbidity and mortality (whether these are caused by infectious agents or other environmental factors, such as carcinogens). These historical and larger-scale social relationships may help us not only to understand AIDS and other epidemics, but also to design interventions to minimize the damage done by the epidemic, and to develop a society that will have mechanisms to cope with future epidemics.

The argument of this paper should not, however, be overstated or misconstrued. Clearly, microsocial and social-psychological theories do serve a valid (although limited) function in explaining and intervening in the epidemic. That is, I am more concerned with the absence of something desirable—namely, an adequately developed sociohistorical awareness to guide our research and actions—than with the presence of something objectionable. Thus, although this paper criticizes the preponderance of microsocial and social-psychological approaches in sociobehavioral AIDS research and in many interventions, I do not dismiss the legitimacy and necessity of such research, nor disparage its usefulness in the tactical, face-to-face aspects of interventions.

Of course, the actual moment of HIV transmission most often occurs during sexual or drug-related activities, which usually involve interaction among only a small group of people (normally two for sex, but sometimes including five or more during drug injection). Obviously, too, in such an interaction, small-group pressures and the psychology of the individual participants play their part—but absent from the now prevailing models of analysis is the understanding that these forces themselves have first been shaped by larger social contexts. For instance, the race and place of residence of the participants, as well as the year in which the event occurs, will affect the probability of whether a virus is even present to transmit. Local policies and laws, as well as cultural factors, help determine whether or not sterile syringes or bleach are present during drug injection. Similarly, the local religion and its legitimacy to participants, as well as economic factors and sociopolitical policies, affect whether condoms are present during sexual activity.

Once these larger contexts are properly factored in, though, microsocial and social-psychological forces remain important. For example, both drug-related (Friedman et al. 1987a) and sexual risk reduction (Abdul-Quader, Tross, Friedman, Kouzi, and Des Jarlais 1990) are more likely among drug injectors whose friends engage in risk reduction, just as risk behavior tends to be lower among drug injectors who maintain close ties with friends, sexual partners, or relatives who do not inject drugs (Neaigus et al. 1990). Abdul-Quader and colleagues (1990) also report that sexual risk reduction is more likely among drug injectors with higher self-efficacy toward avoiding AIDS; perceived present and future susceptibility to HIV infection, however, were not related to sexual risk reduction. Although it should be pointed out that such factors as peer pressure for risk reduction, perceived susceptibility, or even self-efficacy are themselves social products, often resulting from the interaction between subcultures and the larger society, these variables are at the same time microsocial as well.

Nevertheless, as a counterbalancing corrective to the prevailing approaches, this paper will stress the argument that sociohistorical factors have been demonstrably important in the course of the AIDS epidemic. My argument does not rest on any single study but is rather a synthesis based on an extensive body of literature and research. Much of this material is based on work by the author and others in the field of AIDS among drug injectors and their sexual partners, although other materials are drawn upon as well. The focus of this paper is of necessity primarily on the United States, and secondarily on other developed countries. Occasional references are also made to other countries such as Brazil and Thailand but, unfortunately, the available research in developing countries remains insufficient for their experiences to be adequately represented in my analysis. Hence, for example, AIDS in Africa is not addressed, although the work of Charles Hunt (1989) shows the importance of historical and social factors in the spread of AIDS there.

AIDS AS HISTORICALLY SITUATED

AIDS was first announced in an article in *Mortality and Morbidity Weekly Report* in 1981/(Centers for Disease Control 1991)—the first year of the Reagan presidency, early in Margaret Thatcher's period as Prime Minister. It was a period when the priorities of most governments in the industrially developed world focused on confronting intensified international competition, both economic and military, a goal to be achieved partly through drastic cutbacks in social-welfare expenditure. Meanwhile, medical costs continued to rise rapidly throughout the 1980s (even aside from AIDS-related expenditures), so considerable attention was paid to finding ways to reduce this perceived drain on the solvency of governments and the profitability of private enterprises.

These trends were especially noticeable in urban America, where a prolonged period of economic and social retrenchment had begun in the mid-1970s with the New York City "fiscal crisis." The social services offered to the unemployed and the working poor were being cut even as living standards continued to decline, while many low- to moderate-income people were displaced from previously affordable housing, stable neighborhoods, and social networks by "desertification" (Wallace 1990) or gentrification. Through the conjoined impact of these and other factors, New York and other cities saw an increase in long-term poverty among many residents—particularly among racial minorities.

Throughout this period, too, a gradual shift took place in the prevailing perception of urban poverty: from a widely shared optimism regarding the problem-solving potential of an expanding economy (such as had characterized Kennedy's New Frontier and Johnson's Great Society), to a pessimism regarding seemingly intractable social problems. This growing social pessimism was manifest in the deepening despair in poor and working-class communities, which may have increased the supply both of personnel and of customers for the illegal drug trade. Moreover, in the absence of mass popular movements expressing alternative ideas and necessities, political and economic leaders were able to promote a general spirit of blaming the poor for their impoverishment, an attitude that became increasingly prominent in media and as a fashionable ethos of middle-class life. This confluence of events made it feasible for conservative political leaders to gain support for a politics of "social issues" in which they diverted attention from other causal factors by blaming the drug addict and the pushers for the ongoing deterioration of urban life.

Furthermore, this was a period marked by relatively low levels of popular insurgency. The mass movements among blacks, Puerto Ricans, Mexican-Americans/Chicanos, rank-and-file workers, and women had subsided and been replaced by more traditional pluralist electoral and lobbying strategies, together with some efforts to promote social-service agencies and/or profit-making corporations based on these constituencies.

One major exception to this picture of movement quiescence was among gays and lesbians—and even here, the late 1970s marked a retreat from street confrontations and revolutionary aspirations. Instead, there had developed considerable gay influence through a pluralist political approach of influence and voting; an above-ground network of gay retail establishments, newspapers, and other institutions; and a continuing ability to take to the streets in gay pride marches or in reaction to particular attacks upon gay or lesbian rights (Adam 1987).

Thus, when AIDS became a large-scale and visible threat, gays already had an organizational basis in place for a prompt, effective response (Adam 1987;

Altman 1986; Coutinho, Godfried, van Griensven, and Moss 1989; Patton 1985). In contrast, drug injectors in the United States were unorganized (unlike in the Netherlands, as described in de Jong [1986] and in Friedman, de Jong and Des Jarlais [1988]) and were prime scapegoats for a severe moralistic political attack that led to congressional and executive refusal not only to fund syringe exchanges, but even to allow federal funds to be used in research about syringe exchanges.

Unfortunately, this opposition to programs aimed at helping drug injectors protect themselves (and their sexual partners and unborn children) against AIDS received considerable support from some African-American political, religious, and community leaders in cities such as New York, on the basis that such programs putatively encouraged drug use and detracted from drug-abuse treatment budgets. Yet in other cities, such as Baltimore and New Haven, black leaders were more open to research showing that syringe exchanges lack harmful effects and encourage risk reduction, and thus supported these programs.

In other countries, such as the Netherlands or even Margaret Thatcher's Britain, a harm-reduction approach became the basis for AIDS interventions among drug injectors. In the Netherlands, furthermore, there was a willingness to accept the legitimacy and, indeed, desirability of participation by representatives of drug injectors as well as of gays on commissions to develop AIDS policies.

In the United States, however, the lack of a large-scale mass movement in black and Puerto Rican communities, together with the great level of economic distress in many minority neighborhoods, meant that it was not until many years after AIDS became widespread in these neighborhoods that local groups mounted organized responses to the epidemic (Quimby and Friedman 1989). Even then, these first initiatives were met with an at-best ambivalent response from many established local agencies and institutions such as churches, drug-abuse treatment centers, and clinics, which were were devoting most of their attention to maintaining preexisting services in a period of cutbacks, and to promoting noncontroversial behavioral patterns. AIDS risk reduction, with its candid approach to difficult moral issues around sexual and drug-related behavior, was sometimes seen as posing a threat to institutional survival by groups who were materially dependent upon federal funding or voluntary contributions. Also, in many cases, staff were simply too overwhelmed by their other duties to be able to address this new issue.

Nonetheless, the overall conjuncture of historical forces at the time when AIDS first emerged as a serious epidemic did present one somewhat positive aspect: namely, that the historical advance of biomedical science had by then made it possible to identify HIV as an infectious agent, and to study the impact of HIV on the immune system, the central nervous system, and other parts of the body. This, in turn, enabled researchers to develop tests for HIV infection and to use these tests for screening blood to prevent transmission during transfusions. It also allowed the development of medicines that might retard or reverse HIV infection, as well as others to address opportunistic infections such as *pneumocystis carinii pneumonia.* Although the socioeconomic organization of medical research posed serious problems—and, indeed, sparked considerable mass mobilization among gays and others to broaden access to new medicines—the particular developmental level attained by medical science has been an important aspect of the AIDS epidemic. It could be characterized, perhaps, as an epidemic that fell just at the edge of what could be addressed by current scientific knowledge—but also by the fact that the resulting medical regimens were too expensive for the poor in the United States to afford, much less for infected persons (or even entire medical delivery systems) in Central Africa, East Africa, Brazil, Thailand, and other less developed areas of the world.

In summary, then, we can see that there are indeed historical components of the AIDS epidemic. If it had occurred in the mid-1960s, for example, gays would not yet have been organized; a mass black movement would still have existed; the social, political, and economic priorities of policymakers would have been shaped by a different set of forces; and the medical system would have been technologically much less prepared to handle AIDS. If it had not happened until the year 2010, on the other hand, it is unknowable what mix of technical and social dynamics would have been in place.

LOCAL EPIDEMICS ARE SOCIOHISTORICALLY SITUATED

There is considerable inter-area variation in the seroprevalence curves for HIV among drug injectors. Figure 1 presents epidemic curves for New York, San Francisco, Bangkok, Sardinia, and Rio de Janeiro. Two facts leap from this figure. First, the most important single factor in determining whether a drug injector would be infected in one of these cities in 1980 (before AIDS was discovered) was where he or she lived. Drug injectors whose own behaviors, and those of their friends, were of extremely high risk in Bangkok or San Francisco were nonetheless unlikely to be infected at that time, whereas 40 percent of drug injectors in southern Manhattan already were infected.

Second, the slopes of the curves vary. It took two to three years for New York to go from 10 percent seropositive to 40 percent, but it took Bangkok only eight months to do so; and San Francisco has stabilized at about 15 percent for several years. Although we do not fully understand the causes of these differences, they seem unlikely to be because of differences in health beliefs or self-efficacy. (For example, New York saw a slower spread of HIV than Bangkok, but drug injectors in New York could hardly have been aware of AIDS before it was discovered.) Instead, differences in the social structures

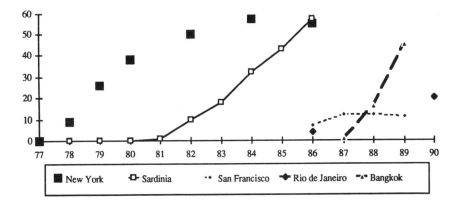

Sources: Bangkok and San Francisco: Stimson (1990); New York: Des Jarlais et al. (1989a); Rio de Janeiro: Bastos, Lima, Lopes, and Dias (1988; and unpublished data) Sardinia: Farci et al. (1988).

Figure 1. Percentage of Drug Injectors Who are Seropositive, by Year

of drug use and/or in public-health policy more probably account for these differences.

Some relevant social-structural differences in these cases might include: (1) the greater presence, and the less private nature, of shooting galleries in New York City in 1975-1985 than in San Francisco, which would have enabled the rapid spread of HIV across friendship groups; (2) possible differences in the speed of gentrification or destruction of neighborhoods (Wallace 1990) that might disperse nuclei of infected drug injectors to spread HIV through continuing their normal injection practices with new persons in their new neighborhoods; or (3) features of the Bangkok jail and prison system that may have allowed for rapid spread among drug injectors who were incarcerated (Vanichseni et al. 1989).

Public-health policies also differ among cities. Amsterdam has acted aggressively against AIDS among drug injectors (and its seroprevalence level has remained relatively stable in the 30 percent range since 1986, as reported by van Haastrecht, van den Hoek, Bardoux, Leentvaar-Kuypers, and Coutinho [1991]). It offers a wide variety of drug-treatment agencies—including methadone buses that travel among areas with large drug-user populations—which vary in the degree to which they regulate and monitor client behaviors; an openness toward organizations that include drug users as part of the policy-making process and even toward drug users' own organizations (although these have been less successful in Amsterdam than the *junkiebonden* in some other Dutch cities such as Rotterdam); and a wide network of syringe exchanges that have been distributing over 700,000 syringes per year (for an estimated drug-injecting population of two to three thousand) for the past several years (Hartgers, Buning, van Santen, Verster, and Coutinho 1989; van den Hoek 1990).

San Francisco's drug-user-oriented AIDS policies have been shaped by the fact that AIDS developed early and massively among its large and influential gay male population, but was much slower to reach its drug injectors. Thus, there was time for social researchers in the city to develop a well-conceived intervention prior to the extensive spread of HIV among the approximately 15,000 drug injectors in the city. They developed an outreach approach that combined ethnographic knowledge of drug-using networks with education and the distribution of bleach and condoms by street-wise outreach workers. Although there have been conflicts among the agencies engaged in these efforts, they have nonetheless been able to build it into a fairly large-scale effort (with perhaps 50 outreach workers, or one-per-300 drug injectors.) In addition, an underground needle-exchange project was established in San Francisco in 1988 that has been distributing more than 5,000 syringes per month (Dietrick 1990). This project, Prevention Point, has won de facto recognition and support from city health and law-enforcement authorities, although technically it remains banned under state law.

New York drug injectors began changing their behaviors to reduce their AIDS risks well before the establishment of any outreach or other projects (Friedman, Des Jarlais, Sotheran, Garber, Cohen, and Smith, 1987; Kleinman, Goldsmith, Friedman, Hopkins, and Des Jarlais 1990; Selwyn, Feiner, Cox, Lipshutz, and Cohen 1987). Two outreach projects began during 1985 and 1986. ADAPT (the Association for Drug Abuse Prevention and Treatment) organized volunteer outreach to conduct education and distribute bleach and condoms in drug-sale areas, even during the several years before paid staff to carry on these activities became available. Narcotic and Drug Research, Inc. received funds from the state health department for outreach, with a primary focus on recruiting drug injectors for HIV-antibody testing and counseling. However, these projects, plus others that have since started up, have never had a staff that totaled even 100 outreach workers combined—while attempting to serve a drug-injecting population of 200,000 or more. That is, the density of outreach workers-to-injectors has been less than one-seventh that in San Francisco. Furthermore, community hostility to drug users has been greater in New York, and opposition to the distribution of bleach has at times been quite strong.

RACIAL STRUCTURE AND THE EPIDEMIC

There is wide variation in AIDS case data by race. Race, of course, is a major element in the American stratification system (Geschwender 1978). Selik,

Castro, and Pappaioanou (1988) have shown that the relative risk of black or Latino adults getting AIDS through any of a wide range of risk behaviors— drug injection, sex with a drug injector, or having a drug injector as a parent, but also (for males) through gay or bisexual behavior—is greater than for whites. (Selik, Castro, and Pappaioanou [1989] also show that Puerto Rican Latinos are more likely to have gotten AIDS than Mexican-American or other Latinos.)

Considerable research has been done on differences in HIV seroprevalence by race among drug injectors. Black and/or Latino IV drug users have higher seropositivity rates than whites in many, although not all, studies (Allen, Onorato, and Sweeney 1989; Brown, Murphy and Primm 1987; Chaisson et al. 1989; Comerford, Chitwood, McCoy, and Trapido 1989; D'Aquila, Peterson, Williams, and William 1989; Des Jarlais and Friedman, 1989b; Friedman, Sotheran, Abdul-Quader, Primm, and Des Jarlais 1987; Hahn, Onorato, Jones, and Dougherty 1989; Lange et al. 1988; Marmor et al. 1987; Novick et al. 1989; Robert-Guroff et al. 1986; Schoenbaum, Selwyn, Hartel, and Friedland 1988; Watters et al. 1989; Weiss et al. 1985). In most studies, race remains a significant predictor even with behavioral controls (Chaisson et al. 1989; D'Aquila, Peterson, Williams, and William 1989; Friedman et al. 1989a; Lewis and Watters 1988.)

Race is also associated with differences in behavioral risk and risk reduction in New York (Friedman, Sotheran, Abdul-Quader, Primm, and Des Jarlais 1987b; Friedman, Sufian, and Des Jarlais 1990; Friedman et al. 1989b; Sufian et al. 1990). White IV drug users had lower drug-injection frequencies than blacks or Latinos in a 1984 treatment sample. Whites also use shooting galleries a smaller percentage of the time than Latinos, both in the 1984 sample and in two later samples of street IV drug users: a treatment sample from the Lower East Side of Manhattan in 1986, and a street-recruited sample from Brooklyn, Queens, and the Bronx in 1988 (Friedman, Sotheran, Abdul-Quader, Primm, and Des Jarlais 1987b; Sufian et al. 1990). White drug injectors in New York also appear to have learned sooner than black or Latino IV drug users about the use of bleach to decontaminate syringes (Friedman, Sotheran, Abdul-Quader, Primm, and Des Jarlais 1987b).

Yet perhaps the most striking research findings are the several studies which indicate that black drug injectors seem to have engaged in greater risk reduction than others. For instance, significantly more Black subjects (48%) than whites (26%) or Latinos (23%) reported that they had reduced sharing works with other IV drug users in order to reduce their risk of getting AIDS (Friedman, Sotheran, Abdul-Quader, Primm, and Des Jarlais 1987b.) Furthermore, a multicity treatment-entrant study (Schober and Schade, 1989) and a San Francisco treatment-entrant study (Woods et al. 1989) find that blacks are less likely to share needles than whites or Hispanics. Finally, a nineteen-city study of street-recruited drug injectors found that blacks are the least likely to borrow used needles or to share cookers or cotton during injection preparations, as well as the most likely to use new needles and, when not doing so, to use alcohol or bleach as a decontaminant (Friedman, Snyder, et al. forthcoming).

Thus, there is a discrepancy between blacks' higher HIV seroprevalence rates and blacks' lesser involvement in risky behaviors. This has yet to be satisfactorily explained. Possible explanations include: blacks having responded more rapidly to the epidemic (but doing so only after many were already infected); racial differences in response biases; different social-network structures that might retard the speed of HIV spread among white drug injectors; and a more extensive, or more frequent, disruption of minority drug-injector networks through gentrification, desertification, or police practices. Differences in social networks or in network disruption clearly call for mid-level or large-scale social structural explanation, and for a more community-oriented and political approach to intervention.

THEORY AND INTERVENTION MODELS

The dominant models of how to prevent the spread of HIV have relied upon psychological and social-psychological models. This has remained so in spite of the fact that the most successful efforts against AIDS have been those of collectively self-organized gay communities and have involved community organizing and the mobilization of group pressure for subcultural change (Bye 1990; Friedman, Des Jarlais, Sotheran, Garber, Cohen, and Smith 1987.) These group efforts have, to be sure, made full use of the insights of psychology and social psychology in designing particular interventions. However, a multifaceted community mobilization has been the key element in recruiting personnel and other resources, and also has produced a context of public concern—achieved only through an often bitter political struggle—about the survival of gay individuals and communities.

Nonetheless, individualistic models have been dominant. For example, in the largest set of interventions to date (the National AIDS Demonstration Research [NADR] and AIDS Targeted Outreach Models [ATOM] established by the National Institute on Drug Abuse in 1987), the underlying models for intervention and (even more) for evaluation were individualistic. Health-education models that viewed risk reduction as the product of individual actors making solitary decisions dominated. Sometimes the probable presence of other actors who might influence drug or sexual behavior was incorporated into the intervention within the parameters of the health-belief model and/ or of social-learning theory. Yet, even here, the focus would usually be on teaching individuals how to negotiate their own risk reduction *as individuals*— rather than on changing group subcultures. Some of the most successful projects, however, used approaches based upon middle-range theories of subcultural adaptation or upon models of group mobilization, rather than relying exclusively upon psychology or small-group social psychology.

As already discussed, San Francisco mounted an outreach model that was based upon ethnographic analyses of the drug subculture and, specifically, of bleach use as an effective innovation that would involve minimal disruption of the established norms, values, and procedures of drug injection (Biernacki and Feldman 1986; Feldman and Biernacki 1988; Newmeyer, Feldman, Biernacki, and Watters 1989; Watters and Biernacki 1989). The San Francisco approach, then, used outreach tools of health education to implement an intervention that acted as a catalyst for further initiatives by those within the drug-using subculture itself, altering their own norms of behavior to adapt to the new threat of HIV.

In Chicago, Wiebel and his colleagues (Wiebel 1988, 1990; Wiebel and Altman 1988; Wiebel, Altman, Chene, and Fritz 1989; Wiebel, Fritz, and Chene 1989) built further upon this approach and designed ways to recruit the outreach-staff individuals who were influential in drug-using neighborhoods and networks. These staff members, furthermore, were under the direct supervision of ethnographers who studied what was happening among local drug users in order to develop appropriate tactics to promote risk reduction. This model, then, involved a merger of ethnography, theory about deviant subcultures, and community-intervention leadership theories.

Finally, at least two projects (in Minneapolis-St. Paul and in New York City) used a community-organizing approach to mobilize drug users against AIDS. Here, the immediate models were those of the gay community and the Dutch *junkiebonden,* but underlying these there were social-movement theories which view community change as the product of organized minorities who pressure from within for risk reduction (Friedman, Des Jarlais, Sotheran, Garber, Cohen, and Smith 1987; Friedman, Sufian, Curtis, Neaigus, and Des Jarlais 1992; Friedman, Neaigus et al. forthcoming; Carlson and Needle, 1989). The New York organizing project had considerable success in promoting risk reduction, including getting up to one-third of the drug injectors in the neighborhood to use condoms consistently when having sex (Jose, Friedman, Neaigus, and Sufian forthcoming).

SOME BRIEF SPECULATIONS ON HEALTH CARE RESEARCH

One of the strong points which proponents have claimed for the health belief model has been its relevance to whether people seek out medical assistance for their problems. Nevertheless, the AIDS epidemic has raised some macrosocial issues about whether persons seek and get access to medical care.

Both gays and drug injectors see themselves, with ample justification, as stigmatized—and thus see getting useful help from social or medical agencies as at best problematic. Gay communities throughout the United States and in many other countries, therefore, have had to respond to the epidemic by pressuring hospitals and clinics to be more accepting of gays, and also by providing their own alternative buddy systems, volunteer clinics, and support groups for the ill, both in hospitals and outside of them. I hypothesize that the probability that a gay man will seek timely medical assistance is largely a function of the degree of such community mobilization in his area; and likewise, that the probability that he will actually receive quality care is also a function of the success of such mobilization.

For drug injectors, the prospect of respectful treatment by hospital staff is even lower. Indeed, in demonstration projects with which I have been associated, I have observed instances of hospitals outright refusing to take drug injectors as patients, as well as of drug injectors finding the way they are treated so unpleasant that they themselves choose to leave, against medical advice. Such experiences provide a rational basis for many drug users to avoid hospitals whenever they can—but this also means that many get treatment too late, if at all. This factor alone is probably a major contributor to the fact that, among drug injectors in New York, HIV-associated mortality from bacterial pneumonia, tuberculosis, endocarditis, and other non-AIDS-defining treatable conditions is as high as AIDS mortality itself (Stoneburner et al. 1988) Where community-based organizations support the users, they are often admitted more easily, and even get more respect.

Of course, these observations about the relationship between gays and/or drug injectors and the medical system need further research to determine their truth and generalizability. If they have broad applicability, however, this would indicate that issues of community mobilization, the strength of stigmas, and perhaps the degree to which medical facilities are adequately staffed and financed are as important, and perhaps more so, than microsocial factors in determining whether the two groups of persons most likely to need AIDS-related medical treatment in the United States seek it, and get it, in timely fashion.

CONCLUSIONS

Many of the most notable features of the AIDS epidemic seem to be historical, macrosocial, or middle-range features of subcultures, rather than microsocial in scope. The microsocial models to which many medical sociologists now limit themselves thus should not remain hegemonic.

In particular, microsociological approaches seem to contribute little to our understanding of who gets AIDS or HIV infection. Disease and seropositivity seem much more to be functions of social and historical factors than of health beliefs or self-efficacy. This may seem obvious, since the microsocial models were never designed to explain infection patterns, but it becomes an important limitation in a period when infectious diseases are again becoming salient.

Furthermore, the extent to which individuals engage in risks or risk reduction also seems to depend heavily on larger structures. A list of some of these large-scale factors would include:

1. Geographical location.
2. Local social structures, including those that shape the ease of spread between gay men and drug injectors, the ease of spread among friendship groups of drug injectors or gay men, and the migration of individuals among such friendship groups.
3. Race, here conceived as an element of social stratification rather than as a personal attribute.
4. Laws, policies, and programs, such as drug-paraphernalia laws, policies toward harm reduction, and funding levels for outreach or organizing projects.

In addition, the risk of getting infected in the United States, Europe, or Australia has so far been heavily dependent upon whether people engage in either or both of two specific behaviors—male-male sex and drug injection. We do not have a good understanding of the causes of either of these behavior patterns. Gay male sexual orientation, however, probably cannot be reduced to a function of the variables highlighted by the health-belief model or social-learning theory. Drug injection may be more readily interpreted in these terms, but also seems to have important components of social class, race, geography (e.g., a far higher proportion of heroin users inject their drugs in the United States than in the Netherlands), and neighborhood subcultures.

Furthermore, individualistic models direct our attention away from the paramount success story of the epidemic to date—the extent to which organized gay communities have been able to reduce HIV transmission and, as well, to provide direct assistance to the sick. This, and the extent to which macrosocial and middle-range models have shaped some of the more successful interventions aimed at drug injectors, point to the importance of looking beyond the individual, and of looking instead at social contexts, and at the macrosocial and historical roots of these social contexts. Unfortunately, AIDS developed as an epidemic in an age when radically individualistic ideologies were politically hegemonic in most of the developed world, and these have characterized an intellectual climate which hinders our ability to develop appropriate theories and interventions to respond to HIV and its effects.

Finally, it is worth ending by highlighting a few questions that this review indicates may be salient ones:

1. Why have the main foci of research and intervention been individualistic? That is, if the analysis presented in this paper is correct, although microsocial approaches are indeed important, the overemphasis on individualism both in medical sociology and in public-health practice should be seen as problematic. Research should be conducted both to understand this overindividualism and to delineate its effects. In overly simple terms, perhaps the individualistic approach is itself a social problem.

2. The gay experience in confronting AIDS, and the contrast between this and the relative lack of collectively organized responses by drug injectors and by minority communities, show the importance of such efforts by communities at risk. This, then, highlights a broader issue for the future: How can we develop a society where self-organization and collective action become easy and normative?

3. What are the social barriers to risk reduction (both group and individual) and to effective public-health measures? What are the social roots of these barriers? What research and practical activity can help remove these barriers and their social roots?

ACKNOWLEDGEMENT

The research in this paper was supported by National Institute on Drug Abuse grant DA06723. The views expressed in this paper do not necessarily reflect the positions of the granting agency or of the institution by which the author is employed.

REFERENCES

Abdul-Quader, A.S., S. Tross, S.R. Friedman, A.C. Kouzi, and D.C. Des Jarlais. 1990. "Street-Recruited Intravenous Drug Users and Sexual Risk Reduction in New York City." AIDS 4: 1075-1079.

Adam, B. 1987. *The Rise of a Gay and Lesbian Movement.* Boston: Twayne.

Allen, D.M., I. Onorato, and P.A. Sweeney. 1989. "Seroprevalence of Human Immunodeficiency Virus Infection in Intravenous Drug Users, United States, 1988-89." Paper presented at the 117th Annual Meeting of the American Public Health Association, Chicago.

Altman, D. 1986. *AIDS in the Mind of America.* Garden City, NY: Doubleday.

Bandura, A. 1977. *Social Learning Theory.* Engelwood, NJ: Prentice-Hall.

Bastos, F.I., E.S. Lima, C.S. Lopes, and P.R.T.P. Dias. 1988. "Perfil de usarios de drogas I. Estudo de caracteristicas de pacientes do NEPAD/UERJ, 1986-87" [Profile of Drug Users I: A Study of the Characteristics of Patients at the NEPAD/UERJ, 1986-87]. *Rev. ABP/APAL* 10: 47-52.

Becker, M.H. and J.K. Joseph. 1988. "AIDS and Behavioral Change To Reduce Risk: A Review." *American Journal of Public Health* 78: 394-410.

Biernacki, P. and H.W. Feldman. 1986. "The Empirical Basis for Preventing the Spread of AIDS among Intravenous Drug Users in San Francisco." Paper presented at the Fifteenth

International Conference on the Prevention and Treatment of Drug Dependence, Amsterdam.

Botvin, G.J., E. Baker, E.M. Botvin, B.S. Filazzola, and R. Millman. 1984. "Prevention of Alcohol Misuse through Development of Personal and Social Competence." *Journal of Studies on Alcohol* 45: 550-552.

Brown, L.S., D.L. Murphy, and B.J. Primm. 1987. "Needle Sharing and AIDS in Minorities." *Journal of the American Medical Association* 258: 1474-1475.

Bye, L.L. 1990. "Moving Beyond Counseling and Knowledge-Enhancing Interventions: A Plea for Community-Level AIDS Prevention Strategies." Pp. 157-170 in *Behavioral Aspects of AIDS*, edited by D.G. Ostrow. New York: Plenum Medical Book Company.

Carlson, G. and R. Needle. 1989. "Sponsoring Addict Self-Organization (Addicts Against AIDS): A Case Study." Paper presented at the First Annual National AIDS Demonstration Research Conference, Rockville, MD.

Centers for Disease Control. 1991. "The HIV/AIDS Epidemic: The First 10 Years." *Morbidity and Mortality Weekly Report* 40: 357-363, 369.

Chaisson, R.E., P. Bacchetti, D. Osmond, B. Brodie, M.A. Sande, and A.R. Moss. 1989. "Cocaine Use and HIV Infection in Intravenous Drug Users in San Francisco." *Journal of the American Medical Association* 261: 561-565.

Comerford, M., D.D. Chitwood, C.B. McCoy, and E.J. Trapido. 1989. "Association Between Former Place of Residence and Serostatus of IVDUs in South Florida." Paper presented at the Fifth International Conference on AIDS, Montreal.

Coutinho, R.A., J.P. Godfried van Griensven, and A. Moss. 1989. "Effects of Preventive Efforts among Homosexual Men." *AIDS* 3 (Supplement 1): S53-S56.

D'Aquila, R.T., L.R. Peterson, A.B. Williams, and A.E. William. 1989. "Race/Ethnicity as a Risk Factor for HIV-1 Infection among Connecticut Intravenous Drug Users." *Journal of Acquired Immune Deficiency Syndromes* 2: 503-513.

de Jong, W.M. 1986. "De sociale beweging van opiatengebruikers in Nederland" ["The Social Relations of Opiate Injectors in the Netherlands"]. Doctoraal-scriiptie sociologie, Erasmus Universiteit, Rotterdam.

Des Jarlais, D.C. and S.R. Friedman. 1988. "The Psychology of Preventing AIDS among Intravenous Drug Users." *American Psychologist* 43: 865-870.

Des Jarlais, D.C. and S.R. Friedman. 1989. "Ethnic Differences in HIV Seroprevalence Rates among IV Drug Users." Pp. 24-33 in *AIDS and Intravenous Drug Abuse among Minorities*, edited by R.W. Pickens. Rockville, MD: National Institute on Drug Abuse.

Des Jarlais, D.C., S.R. Friedman, D.M. Novick, J.L. Sotheran, P. Thomas, S.R. Yancovitz, D. Mildvan, J. Weber, M.J. Kreek, R. Maslansky, S. Bartelme, T. Spira, and M. Marmor. 1989. "HIV-1 Infection among IV Drug Users Entering Treatment in Manhattan, New York City." *Journal of the American Medical Association* 261: 1008-1012.

Dietrick, R. 1990. "Description of San Francisco's Prevention Point." Paper presented at the North American Syringe Exchange Convention. Tacoma, Washington.

Emmons, C.A., J.G. Joseph, R.C. Kessler, C.B. Wortman, S.B. Montgomery, and D.G. Ostrow. 1986. "Psychosocial Predictors of Reported Behavior Change in Homosexual Men At Risk for AIDS." *Health Education Quarterly* 13: 331-345.

Evans, R.J. 1976. "Smoking in Children: Developing a Social Psychological Theory of Deterrence." *Preventive Medicine* 5: 122-127.

Farci, P., D.M. Novick, M.E. Lai, G. Orgiana, A. Strazzera, A., S.T. Beatrice, D.C. Des Jarlais, and A. Balestrieri. 1988. "Introduction of Human Immunodeficiency Virus Infection among Parenteral Drug Abusers in Sardinia: A Seroepidemiologic Study." *American Journal of Epidemiology* 127: 1312-1314.

Feldman, H.W. and P. Biernacki. 1988. "The Ethnography of Needle-Sharing among Intravenous Drug Users and Implications for Public Policies and Intervention Strategies." In *Needle*

Sharing among Intravenous Drug Abusers (National Institute on Drug Abuse, Research Monograph Series, No. 80), edited by R.J. Battjes and R.W. Pickens. Washington: U.S. Department of Health and Human Services.

Friedman, S.R., W.M. de Jong, and D.C. Des Jarlais. 1988. "Problems and Dynamics of Organizing Intravenous Drug Users for AIDS Prevention." *Health Education Research* 3: 49-57.

Friedman, S.R., D.C. Des Jarlais, J.L. Sotheran, J. Garber, H. Cohen, and D. Smith. 1987. "AIDS and Self-Organization among Intravenous Drug Users." *International Journal of the Addictions* 22: 201-219.

Friedman, S.R., A. Neaigus, B. Jose, M. Sufian, B. Stepherson, D. Manthei, P. Mota, and D.C. Des Jarlais. Forthcoming. "Behavioral Outcomes of Organizing Drug Injectors Against AIDS." *Proceedings of the Second National AIDS Demonstration Research Conference.* Rockville, MD: National Institute on Drug Abuse Monograph.

Friedman, S.R., E. Quimby, M. Sufian, A. Abdul-Quader, and D.C. Des Jarlais. 1989. "Racial Aspects of the AIDS Epidemic." *California Sociologist* 11: 55-68.

Friedman, S.R., A. Rosenblum, D. Goldsmith, D.C. Des Jarlais, M. Sufian, and A. Neaigus. 1989. "Risk Factors for HIV-1 Infection among Street-Recruited Intravenous Drug Users in New York City." Paper presented at the Fifth International Conference on AIDS, Montreal.

Friedman, S.R., F.R. Snyder, V. Shorty, A. Jones, A.L. Estrada, and P.A. Young. Forthcoming. "Racial Differences in HIV Risk Behaviors among Drug Injectors: Multicity Data." *Proceedings of the Second National AIDS Demonstration Research Conference.* Rockville, MD: National Institute on Drug Abuse Monograph.

Friedman, S.R., J.L. Sotheran, A. Abdul-Quader, B.J. Primm, D.C. Des Jarlais, P. Kleinman, C. Maugé, D.S. Goldsmith, W. El-Sadr, and R. Maslansky. 1987. "The AIDS Epidemic among Blacks and Hispanics." *The Milbank Quarterly* 65(Supplement 2): 455-499.

Friedman, S.R., M. Sufian, R. Curtis, A. Neaigus, and D.C. Des Jarlais. 1992. "Organizing Drug Users Against AIDS." Pp. 115-130 in *The Social Context of AIDS,* edited by J. Huber and B.E. Schneider. Newbury Park, CA: Sage.

Friedman, S.R., M. Sufian, and D.C. Des Jarlais. 1990. "The AIDS Epidemic among Latino Intravenous Drug Users." Pp. 45-54 in *Drug Use in Hispanic Communities,* edited by R. Glick and J. Moore. New Brunswick, NJ: Rutgers University Press.

Geschwender, J.A. 1978. *Racial Stratification in America.* Dubuqueia: William C. Brown.

Hahn, R.A., I.M. Onorato, T.S. Jones, and J. Dougherty. 1989. "Prevalence of HIV Infection among Intravenous Drug Users in the United States." *Journal of the American Medical Association* 261: 2677-2684.

Hartgers, C., E.C. Buning, G.W. van Santen, A.D. Verster, and R.A. Coutinho. 1989. "The Impact of the Needle and Syringe-Exchange Programme in Amsterdam on Injecting Risk Behavior." *AIDS* 3: 571-576.

Hunt, C.W. 1989. "Migrant Labor and Sexually Transmitted Disease: AIDS in Africa." *Journal of Health and Social Behavior* 30: 353-373.

Jose, B., S.R. Friedman, A. Neaigus, and M. Sufian. Forthcoming. "Condom Use among Drug Injectors in an Organizing Project Neighborhood." *Proceedings of the Second National AIDS Demonstration Research Conference.* Rockville, MD: National Institute on Drug Abuse Monograph.

Kleinman, P.H., D.S. Goldsmith, S.R. Friedman, W. Hopkins, and D.C. Des Jarlais. 1990. "Knowledge About and Behaviors Affecting the Spread of AIDS: A Street Survey of Intravenous Drug Users and Their Associates in New York City." *International Journal of the Addictions* 25: 345-362.

Lange, W.R., F.R. Snyder, D. Lozovsky, V. Kaistha, M.A. Kaczaniuk, and J.H. Jaffe. 1988. "Geographic Distribution of Human Immunodeficiency Virus Markers in Parenteral Drug Abusers." *American Journal of Public Health* 78: 443-446.

Lewis, D.K. and J.K. Watters. 1988. "HIV Seropositivity and IVDUs: Ethnic/Gender Comparisons." *American Journal of Public Health* 78: 1499.

Marmor, M., D.C. Des Jarlais, H. Cohen, S.R. Friedman, S.T. Beatrice, N. Dubin, W. El-Sadr, D. Mildvan, S. Yancovitz, U. Mathur, and R. Holzman. 1987. "Risk Factors for Infection with Human Immunodeficiency Virus among Intravenous Drug Abusers in New York City." *AIDS* 1: 39-44.

Montgomery, S.B., J.G. Joseph, M.H. Becker, D.G. Ostrow, R.C. Kessler, and J.P. Kirscht. 1989. "The Health Belief Model in Understanding Compliance with Preventive Recommendations for AIDS: How Useful?" *AIDS Education and Prevention* 1: 303-323.

Neaigus, A., S.R. Friedman, M. Sufian, B. Stepherson, D.S. Goldsmith, and P. Mota. 1990. "Effects of Peer Culture, Race, and Gender on IV Drug Use Risk Reduction." Paper presented at the 118th Annual Meeting of the American Public Health Association, New York City, October.

Newmeyer, J.A., H.W. Feldman, P. Biernacki, and J.K. Watters. 1989. "Preventing AIDS Contagion among Intravenous Drug Users." *Medical Anthropology* 10: 167-175.

Novick, D.M., H.L. Trigg, D.C. Des Jarlais, S.R. Friedman, D. Vlahov, and M.J. Kreek. 1989. "Cocaine Injection and Ethnicity in Parenteral Drug Users During the Early Years of the Human Immunodeficiency Virus (HIV) Epidemic in New York City." *Journal of Medical Virology* 29: 181-185.

Patton, C. 1985. *Sex and Germs: The Politics of AIDS*. Boston: South End Press.

Quimby, E. and S.R. Friedman. 1989. "Dynamics of Black Mobilization Against AIDS in New York City." *Social Problems* 36: 403-415.

Robert-Guroff, M., S.H. Weiss, J.A. Giron, A.M. Jennings, H.M. Ginzburg, I.B. Margolis, W.A. Blattner, and R.C. Gallo. 1986. "Prevalence of Antibodies to HTLV-I, -II, and -III in Intravenous Drug Abusers from an AIDS Endemic Region." *Journal of the American Medical Association* 225: 3133-3137.

Schober, S.E. and C. Schade. 1989. "Needle Sharing among Addicts Admitted to Treatment." Paper presented at the 117th Annual Meeting of the American Public Health Association, Chicago.

Schoenbaum, E.E., P.A. Selwyn, D. Hartel, and G.H. Friedland. 1988. "HIV Infection in Intravenous Drug Users in New York City: The Relation of Drug Use and Heterosexual Behaviors and Race/Ethnicity." Paper presented at the Fourth International Conference on AIDS, Stockholm.

Selik, R.M., K.G. Castro, and M. Pappaioanou. 1988. "Racial/Ethnic Differences in the Risk of AIDS in the United States." *American Journal of Public Health* 78: 1539-1545.

_____. 1989. "Birthplace and the Risk of AIDS among Hispanics in the United States." *American Journal of Public Health* 79: 836-839.

Selwyn, P.A., C. Feiner, C.P. Cox, C. Lipshutz, and R.L. Cohen. 1987. "Knowledge About AIDS and High-Risk Behavior among Intravenous Drug Users in New York City." *AIDS* 1: 247-254.

Stimson, G.V. 1990. "The Prevention of HIV Infection in Injecting Drug Users: Recent Advances and Remaining Obstacles." Paper presented at the Sixth International Conference on AIDS, San Francisco.

Stoneburner, R.L., D.C. Des Jarlais, D. Benezra, L. Gorelkin, J.L. Sotheran, S.R. Friedman, S. Schultz, M. Marmor, D. Mildvan, and R. Maslansky. 1988. "A Larger Spectrum of Severe HIV-Related Disease in Intravenous Drug Users in New York City." *Science* 242: 916-919.

Sufian, M., S.R. Friedman, A. Neaigus, B. Stepherson, J. Rivera-Beckman, and D.C. Des Jarlais. 1990. "Impact of AIDS on Puerto Rican Intravenous Drug Users." *Hispanic Journal of Behavioral Sciences* 12: 122-134.

van den Hoek, J.A.R. 1990. *Epidemiology of HIV Infection among Drug Users in Amsterdam.*
    Amsterdam: Rodopi.
van Haastrecht, H.J.A., J.A.R. van den Hoek, C. Bardoux, A. Leentvaar-Kuypers, and R.A.
    Coutinho. 1991. "The Course of the HIV Epidemic among Intravenous Drug Users in
    Amsterdam, The Netherlands." *American Journal of Public Health* 81: 59-62.
Vanichseni, S., N. Wright, P. Akarasewi, W. Pokapanichwong, D. Taylor, and K. Choopanya.
    1989. "Case Control Study of HIV Positivity among Male Intravenous Drug Addicts
    (IVDA) in Bangkok." Paper presented at the Fifth International Conference on AIDS,
    Montreal.
Wallace, R. 1990. "Urban Desertification, Public Health and Public Order: 'Planned Shrinkage',
    Violent Death, Substance Abuse and AIDS in the Bronx." *Social Science and Medicine*
    31: 801-813.
Watters, J.K. and P. Biernacki. 1989. "Targeted Sampling: Options for the Study of Hidden
    Populations." *Social Problems* 36: 416-430.
Watters, J.K., Y.-T. Cheng, J.R. Carlson, P.L. Case, J. Lorvick, K.H.C. Huang, and S.B. Shade.
    1989. "Challenges in Modeling HIV Infection in Low Prevalence Populations." Paper
    presented at the Fifth International Conference on AIDS, Montreal.
Weiss, S.H., H.M. Ginzburg, J.J. Goedert, R.J. Biggar, B.A. Mohica, and W.A. Blattner. 1985.
    "Risk for HTLV-III Exposure among Parenteral Drug Abusers in New Jersey." Paper
    presented at the First International Conference on AIDS, Atlanta, GA.
Wiebel, W. 1988. "Combining Ethnographic and Epidemiologic Methods for Targeted AIDS
    Interventions: The Chicago Model." Pp. 137-150 in *Needle Sharing Among Intravenous
    Drug Abusers: National and International Perspectives,* Research Monograph No. 80.
    Rockville, MD: National Institute on Drug Abuse.
————. 1990. "Identifying and Gaining Access to Hidden Populations." In *The Collection and
    Interpretation of Data from Hidden Populations,* Research Monograph No. 98. Rockville,
    MD: National Institute on Drug Abuse.
Wiebel, W. and N. Altman, 1988. "AIDS Prevention Outreach to IVDUs in Four U.S. Cities."
    Paper presented at the 4th International Conference on AIDS, Stockholm.
Wiebel, W., N. Altman, D. Chene. and R. Fritz. 1989. "Risk Taking and Risk Reduction among
    IV Drug Users in 4 U.S. Cities." Paper presented at the Fifth International Conference
    on AIDS, Montreal.
Wiebel, W., R. Fritz, and D. Chene. 1989. "Description of Intervention Procedures Utilized by
    the AIDS Outreach Intervention Projects—University of Illinois at Chicago, School of
    Public Health." Pp. 68-79 in *Proceedings of the Community Epidemiology Work Group:
    Chicago–June 1989.* Rockville, MD: National Institute on Drug Abuse.
Woods, W.J., A. Abramowitz, J. Guydish, W. Clark, N. Hearst, and R. Kiefer. 1989 "Predicting
    Needle-Sharing Behavior of IVDUs in Treatment." Paper presented at the Fifth
    International Conference on AIDS, Montreal.

RISK PERCEPTIONS AND AIDS

Jennie Jacobs Kronenfeld, Deborah C. Glik,

and Kirby Jackson

ABSTRACT

This paper explores risk perceptions of AIDS, focusing upon two dimensions
of likelihood and seriousness. It draws conceptually upon previous lines of
research in perceptions of risk. While the major focus is on perceptions of AIDS,
some brief comparisons are made to other health problems. Data are available
from a random digit-dial telephone survey of the adult population of four counties
in South Carolina in the fall of 1989 ($N = 628$ households). Most people in this
sample perceive themselves to be at no risk of contracting AIDS within the next
five years. Such a perception is unlikely to create a positive climate towards
behavior changes or attention to discussions about AIDS. People do discriminate
between likelihood of developing AIDS versus other health problems, since
contraction or development of other health problems are all seen as much more
likely. Almost everyone perceived AIDS as extremely serious. Age, sex,
education, marital status, urban/rural location and some AIDS behavior
variables are significant predictors of one's estimate of likelihood of contracting
AIDs and the multiplicative function of likelihood times seriousness. Age and
sex are the only significant predictors of seriousness of AIDS. As treatment for

The Social and Behavioral Aspects of AIDS.
Advances in Medical Sociology, Volume 3, pages 37-57.
Copyright © 1993 by JAI Press Inc.
All Rights of reproduction in any form reserved.
ISBN: 1-55938-439-5

AIDS improves, there will be more variability in how seriously AIDS is viewed, making the multiplicative function more useful. The multiplicative analyses help to point out the importance of rural-urban location as one demographic predictor which has received little attention in previous studies.

INTRODUCTION

This paper reports on research concerning measures of perceived risk of AIDS. The development of the measures draws on a body of knowledge in cognitive psychology. This paper applies the concept of perceived risk to various illness conditions, focusing particularly on AIDS. In the cognitive psychology literature, perceptions of risk are conceptualized not only as how likely or probable it is that a person will develop a problem, but how serious the problem is. This paper explores whether it is useful to include the severity dimension in assessing perceptions of risk of AIDS. Variability in perceptions of risk of AIDS is also examined, focusing on such explanatory groupings as demographic variables, health variables, and AIDS-specific variables. One additional contribution of this study to the AIDS literature is a focus on perceptions of AIDS with explicit rural-urban comparisons, although within the context of a state with relatively low rates of AIDS at the time of the study.

PERCEPTIONS OF RISK

The notion of probabilistic risks of populations in regard to disease has been a major contribution of epidemiologists to our understanding of health and illness in the twentieth century. Given the widespread dissemination of the notion of "risk factors" to at least the educated lay public as part of the discussion of heart disease or cancer risks, most people are now able to discuss whether certain actions are risky and whether there are factors about their own background, genetics, general lifestyle, or specific behaviors which will make them more likely to develop certain diseases or health problems (Slovic 1987; Fischoff, Slovic, and Lichenstein 1978).

Many different disciplines discuss the concept of risk. In epidemiology, the concept of risk factors has been discussed for over 30 years. The approach within epidemiology (and particularly preventive medicine as it has developed) focuses upon "real" risks and an emphasis on understanding factors which help to predict the development of a disease.

The origins of the perceived-risk construct are in the fields of psychology, business, and economics (Tversky and Kahneman 1974; Kahneman and Tversky 1982). Beginning in the 1970s, economists, psychologists and risk analysts began to discuss distinctions between "real" risk and "perceived" risk.

Measurement of real risk assumes that risk is an omnipresent, mathematically measurable possibility of harm that applies to natural events as well as to human actions (Thompson 1990). Early research on risk was dominated by expected utility theory, that is that people make decisions based on rational assessments of outcome probabilities according to some set of commonly accepted inferential principles. This normative view—in which persons acted as "intuitive scientists"—did not hold up in actual descriptive and experimental studies (Nisbett and Ross 1980).

Perceived risk includes a subjective component and thus not only considers outcome probabilities, but also assigns a value to the potential losses and gains of an outcome (Kahneman and Tversky 1979b). This assignment causes decision making to become a function of inconsistent preferences. Even if science (such as epidemiology) can provide us with real risk-probabilities, knowledge of real risk is only one factor in decision making for the lay person. Subjective perceptions or perceived risks reflect the interpretation of scientifically derived knowledge into personal terms. It is this subjective assessment of disease risk that can legitimately be called perceived risk (Fischoff, Slovic, and Lichtenstein 1978).

Kahneman and Tversky (1979a) have shown that there are certain cognitive "heuristics" that people use in determining risk that result in systematic biases. For example, people tend to overestimate the probability of rare but serious events and underestimate the probability of common but less serious events. Many people are very optimistic about their individual chances of avoiding risk (Slovic, Fischoff, and Lichenstein 1977).

Interest in this construct of perceived risk has been growing in many areas of research. The construct is very important to the burgeoning area of inquiry known as risk assessment and risk communications (Wildavsky 1982; Davies, Covello, and Allen 1987; National Research Council 1989). Risk perception has also become the subject of a growing body of research with more traditional sociological roots (Douglas 1985; Nelkin 1989; Szasz 1988). In much of this work, social-structural and cultural differences constitute the grounds for misperception, miscommunication, and outright conflict between different social groups.

The perception of risk area is broader than medical sociology or health services research. Within health-related research, however, in addition to the intellectual interest in understanding differences between real risks and how people perceive risks, people's perceptions of whether they are at risk for certain health problems is increasingly considered critical in explaining why people engage in health-related behaviors or make decisions about the use of health care services. Within health education and in behavior-change programs, there is interest in the similarities between the construct of perceived risk and the idea of perceived susceptibility which is part of the health belief model, the most widely used model of health behavior within health education (Becker 1974; Janz and Becker 1984; Becker and Janz 1987).

One specific development of the perceived-risk concept within psychology has integrated constructs from behavioral decision theory, the health belief model, and the theory of reasoned action as well as from classical social-learning theory. In Weinstein's (1980, 1982) initial development of the precaution adoption process, he found that persons tend to adopt an optimistic bias toward health risks, minimizing or underestimating true risks. This optimistic bias has been confirmed in some studies of cardiovascular disease (Becker and Levine 1987; Niknian, McKinlay, Rakowski, and Carleton 1988).

Weinstein (1982) and Kahneman and Tversky (1979) emphasize that perceived risk is more than the perceived chance you will have a certain outcome by a certain time period. There is also a subjective rating of how serious the unwanted outcome is, leading to the need to include two dimensions, those of likelihood and seriousness, in the development of perceptions of risk. In more recent work, Weinstein (1987) has developed a multi stage theory of health-protective behavior that includes knowledge of risks or hazards, beliefs that protective actions are effective, and belief that one's own actions can make a difference in one's own risk profile. Drawing upon this approach as well as our own work on child safety, we have suggested that the perception of risk to a health problem can be viewed mathematically as the product of perceived likelihood (chances) times perceived seriousness (Kronenfeld and Glik 1991; Kronenfeld, Glik, and Jackson 1991; Glik, Kronenfeld, and Jackson forthcoming).

PERCEPTIONS OF RISK OF AIDS

The epidemic of AIDS with its dismal prognosis and stringent behavioral precautions, has spurred a great deal of research that addresses cognition and behavioral characteristics of people. The construct of perceived risk of AIDS has been receiving attention in the research literature and in federal surveys relating to AIDS. Before attitudes about risk perception and AIDS can be assessed, people must have some understanding and knowledge of the risk (disease) so that they are able to form subjective interpretations. Almost all studies show that now virtually everyone has heard of AIDS (Albrecht, Levy, Sugrue, Prohaska, and Ostrow 1989). Between 1983 and 1986, the percentage of the population who personally knew someone with AIDS doubled up to six percent and continues to increase (Singer, Roger, and Corcoran 1987). Also, most studies now show that most people know that AIDS leads to death, that there is no cure, and that AIDS is transmitted by sexual contact (Dawson and Thornberry 1988; Dawson 1990). Thus, most people should feel capable of responding to questions about their perceived risk of AIDS.

Many surveys have been conducted examining attitudes toward AIDS, including over 20 nationwide surveys conducted as part of public opinion surveys and the provision of special questions in state surveys conducted by the Centers for Disease Control (CDC) as part of the Behavioral Risk Factor Surveillance system (Singer, Roger, Corcoran 1987). In addition, the National Center for Health Statistics (NCHS) has collected data on AIDS knowledge and attitudes (Dawson and Thornberry 1988; Dawson and Hardy 1989; Dawson 1990).

Some of these national surveys as well as a number of smaller surveys in special locations have asked questions relating to risk for AIDS, psychosocial determinants of AIDS, and behaviors which place a person at greater risk for AIDS (McKusick, Horstman, and Coates 1985; Stall, McKusick, Wiley, Coates, and Ostrow 1986; Marin 1989; Windle 1989; Cleary, Rogers, Singer, Avorn, Van Devanter, Perry, and Pindyck 1986; Nelkin 1989, Becker and Joseph 1988). A number of behavioral dimensions have emerged as important to monitor; the number of sexual partners within the past year, adherence to norms of safe sex, and use of condoms are the most important. Other studies have explored fear and social anxiety in terms of public attitudes toward people with AIDS (Thompson 1987; Bean, Keller, Newburg, and Brown 1989). In addition, a number of studies have now been conducted that look at the psychosocial determinants of AIDS-related behaviors (Emmons, Joseph, Kessler, Wortman, Montgomery, and Ostrow 1986; Joseph, Montgomery, Emmons, Kessler, Ostrow, Wortman, O'Brien, Eller, and Eshleman 1987; Neubauer 1989; Kelley et al. 1989, Prohaska, Albrecht, Levy, Sugrue, and Kim 1990).

Several related approaches have been used to ask people whether they consider themselves to be at risk for AIDS. The National Center for Health Statistics has been asking people to rate the chances that they or someone they know may have been infected with HIV, with the responses being high, medium, low, or none (Dawson and Thornberry 1988; Dawson and Hardy 1989; Dawson 1990). In the 1990 data, 81 percent of respondents thought there was no chance of their having been infected with AIDS, 15 percent thought there was a low chance; and two and one percent thought there was a medium or high chance respectively of already being infected. Between the last quarter of 1989 and the first quarter of 1990, the proportion of persons who thought there was no chance of their becoming infected with AIDS dropped from 77 to 73 percent (Dawson 1990). While these questions deal with risk for AIDS, they are not that similar to the perceived-risk construct.

Several recent articles have looked more explicitly at perception of risk (Becker and Joseph 1988; Prohaska, Albrecht; Levy, Sugrue, and Kim 1990; Allard 1989; McKuser, Zapka, Stoddard, and Mayer 1989; Emmons, Joseph, Kessler, Wortman, Montgomery, and Ostrow 1986; Joseph et al. 1987). The focus of some of these articles has been on correlating risk and behavior. Some of the results are contradictory, with two studies reporting a positive correlation between greater perceived risk and behavior change (Allard 1989; McKuser,

Zapka, stoddard, and Mayer 1989) and two others showing no positive correlation between perceptions of risk and behavior (Emmons, Joseph, Kessler, Wortman, Montgomery, and Ostrow 1986; Joseph et al. 1987).

Measurement of perceived risk and the actual emphasis on the attitudinal variables also differs from study to study. In some of these articles, the perceived-risk variable is based on the perceived susceptibility of acquiring an illness (Becker 1974; Becker and Joseph 1988; Allard 1989). Others focused on perceived susceptibility, with questions dealing with whether people were afraid of getting AIDS and if they felt they were more likely to get AIDS than other people (DiClimente, Boyer, and Morales 1988; Taylor-Nicholson, Wang, and Adame 1989). In one study among adolescents, respondents answered questions related to perceived threat such as that AIDS is a health scare taken seriously and that AIDS is the scariest disease known (Koopman, Rotheram-Borus, Henderson, Bradley, and Hunter 1990). In a study of another specialized group, gay men, respondents were asked to describe their own risk of acquiring AIDS and compare it to other gay men (Emmons, Joseph, Kessler, Wortman, Montgomery, and Ostrow 1986).

A study most similar to our own work concentrated on perceived chances of acquiring AIDS in a general population in metropolitan Chicago (Prohaska, Albrecht, Levy, Sugrue, and Kim 1990). In that study, people were asked whether, in terms of their own risk of getting AIDs, they thought they were at great risk, at some risk or at no risk. For analytical purposes, all answers were grouped into two categories of no perceived risk and some or great risk together. Eight different variables were statistically significant predictors of perception of risk: being Asian, having no religious preference, number of sexual partners, knowledge of sexual partners' sexual habits, change in lifestyle as a protective action in response to AIDS, fear of AIDS, how much respondents worry about their health, and shame in contracting AIDS (Prohaska, Albrecht, Levy, Sugrue, and Kim 1990). Demographic variables relating to higher epidemiological risk for AIDS, such as being male and single, were not associated with greater perception of risk. Our study employed a similar question on perceived chances in a general population but added the dimension of severity.

METHODS

Data Collection and Sample

A random digit dial telephone survey was used to collect these data. The methodology for these types of studies is now well established and the phone survey followed procedures recommended by experts and the National Center for Health Statistics on variation in calls by day of week and number of attempted phone calls before abandoning a number (Frey 1983; Groves and Kahn 1979; Groves 1989). About five percent of telephone interviews were verified by a survey supervisor to provide quality control over the data-collection effort.

Four counties in South Carolina, two urban ones which together comprise the metropolitan area, and two rural ones adjacent to the two urban counties were the focus of this study. One goal of the project was to aid the state health department in estimating attitudes toward and behavior related to AIDs in rural and urban South Carolina. Thus, the sampling frame was constructed to obtain a similar number of interviews (about 300) in the two groups of counties (urban versus rural). In each county, lists of eligible telephone exchanges were obtained from the local telephone companies. Using these lists, random telephone numbers were generated and supplied to the interviewers. Thus, the sample is representative of each county grouping but is not proportional to the actual population distribution in the two rural versus two urban counties.

From an initial list of phone numbers, about 83 percent were discarded due to being businesses, disconnected, or always ringing as busy, or not answered after over five attempts. In addition, in 49 cases interviewers reached a household but were told no eligible respondent (an adult 18 or over) resided there. Complete refusals to participate occurred in 66 households. The response rate, computed as the proportion of interviews obtained in all households in which a person was contacted, was 618 of 789 households, or 78 percent. On all basic demographic variables, the urban respondents in the completed telephone survey were almost identical to the census population statistics for the metropolitan area, and the rural respondents were very similar to average census statistics for the two rural counties.

Measurement

Many aspects of the questionnaire used in this study were an adaptation of prior studies with college students (Diclemete, Zorn, and Temoshok 1986) and the general public (Dawson and Thornberry 1988). This was particularly true of questions about practices which place a person at higher risk for AIDS, AIDS knowledge items, and questions on sources of information about AIDS.

The attitudinal questions, especially those relating to perceived risk, included a more detailed attempt to measure perceptions of risk based on conceptual approaches and an adaptation of our own work in child safety (Kronenfeld and Glik 1990; Glik, Kronenfeld, and Jackson 1991). In the perceived-risk literature, there has been an emphasis of perception of risk as having two dimensions, one of likelihood and one of seriousness (Weinstein 1982). We have developed the use of both dimensions in our child safety work (Kronenfeld and Glik 1990; Glik, Kronenfeld, and Jackson 1991) and in this paper are applying the approach to AIDS. In this study, people were asked about both the dimensions of chances (likelihood) and seriousness. For the likelihood or chances item, people were asked to rate the chances in the next five years that they would develop AIDS on a scale from 1 = no chance at all, 2 = extremely unlikely, 3 = fairly likely, 4 = unlikely, 5 = fairly likely, 6 = extremely likely, and 7 = already have the disease. The seriousness dimension asking people how serious they felt AIDS was on a scale from 1 = not serious to 5 = very serious. To allow some comparison between AIDS and other diseases, the AIDS questions on chances and seriousness were asked as part of a series of questions about relatively major chronic health problems (heart problems, high blood pressure, and cancer), relatively minor health problems (having poison oak or ivy, and having a sore throat), and about one major and one relatively minor type of injury (a serious car accident and cutting oneself enough to need stitches). In addition, chances and seriousness can be viewed as separate but related dimensions of perceptions of risk. Thus, it was useful to combine these two dependent variables in some way. A multiplicative construct of the two dimensions of perceived risk of AIDS has also been created. These three perceived risk-of-AIDS variables (chances, seriousness and multiplicative function) are the major ones examined in this paper.

The major independent variables examined were social and demographic variables, general health-status variables, and AIDS-specific variables for the examination of the perceptions of risk of AIDS. Sociodemographic variables included age, sex, race, marital status, urban/rural location, education, and income. Three questions were asked relating to self-perceived health status. Two of these were the commonly used items of self-rate of health from excellent to poor and worry about health from a great deal to none. The third health-related variable was an estimate of energy level compared to others, as adapted from the Alameda county studies (Belloc, Breslow, and Hochstim 1971; Berkman and Breslow 1983). In addition, a number of questions specific to AIDS and sexual behavior were asked. These included items designed to determine patterns of homosexual behavior, use of condoms and types of intercourse, number of sexual partners in the past year, knowledge items about AIDS similar to those used by recent federal surveys, and questions on sources of information about AIDS (Dawson and Thornberry 1988).

Analysis

After an initial examination of frequency distributions for the basic demographic, health, and AIDS variables, as well as the perceptions of risk variables, logistic-regression analysis was used to examine the multiple contribution of variation by three different types of factors—social and demographic factors, health factors and AIDS-specific factors. Three sets of regression analyses were performed, with the different perceptions of AIDS—

dependent variables—perceived seriousness of AIDs, perceived severity of AIDS, and a multiplicative function of the two dimensions. In preliminary work, models utilizing the full scales on the perceptions of risk variables were initially employed, but further examination indicated that the dichotomous-perception variables were more appropriate given the distributions of the perceived risk of AIDS variables in this study. Once dichotomous-dependent variables were being examined, logistic-regression techniques rather than standard multiple-regression techniques were more appropriate. For the logistic analyses, first all social, demographic, and health variables were examined as one group of explanatory factors. Then AIDS-related variables were examined separately. Lastly, comprehensive models were developed for each dependent perceptual variable which included the specific AIDS items as well as the more general social, demographic, and health-related items. The results from these comprehensive models were confirmed using a step-wise logistic-regression analysis.

RESULTS

Demographic, Health, and AIDS-Specific Characteristics

The sample population was very similar to the census characteristics of the sampled counties and basic demographic characteristics are contained in Table 1. The population was almost evenly split in education between those with a high school degree or less and those with at least some college education. About two-thirds of the sample was white and one-third was black. The proportion of females was almost 60 percent, as was the proportion currently married. About 40 percent of the sample were in the 20,000 to 29,999 income group and about the same percentage earned 30,000 or more. Lastly, as planned by the design of the study, about half (51%) of the sample were urban and the rest rural.

Self-reported health characteristics are also presented in Table 1. Overall, this was a relatively healthy population. About three-quarters of the sample perceived their health as excellent or good. Only six percent perceived it as fair. The sample splits into about 45 percent each who worry some or none about their health, leaving only 11 percent with a great deal of worry. In terms of energy level, 40 percent felt they had more energy than others, and about 47 percent felt they had the same amount. There were in each of the indicators, however, enough of a group who may be those with health problems to see whether variation in these health measures influenced perceptions of risk for the different types of health-related problems.

Sexual practices related to AIDS should particularly be important in a person's estimate of his or her own risk for AIDS, while they should be less

Table 1.   Basic Demographic Characteristics of the Survey Group

	Percent
Education	
Less than 12	16.0
High School Graduate	35.04
Some College	19.6
College Graduate	29.1
Race	
White	67.3
Black	32.7
Other	1.0
Gender	
Male	40.3
Female	59.7
Income	
Less then 20,000	17.8
20,000 - 29,999	40.5
30,000		41.6
Area of Residence	
Urban	50.8
Rural	49.2
Self Rate of Health	
Excellent	28.4
Good	53.4
Fair	12.4
Poor	5.9
Worry About Health	
A Great Deal	10.9
Some	46.1
None	43.0
Comparison of Energy with Others	
A Lot More	7.4
Somewhat More	33.2
About Average	46.6
Somewhat Less	9.9
A Lot Less	2.9

important in determination of perceptions of seriousness. On one important question for AIDS research, whether a person had a sexual partner in the past year of the same sex, the numbers reporting such practices were too small for any further analysis. Only 10 women and 15 men reported any sexual partners

Table 2.   Reported Sexual Bahaviors by Gender and Age

| | Percent Reportisng the Given Behavior | | | |
| | Gender* | | Age** | |
Sexual Pracstices	Male	Female	Under 30	30 and Over
Number of Sexual Partners				
0	17.3	34.9	17.1	30.6
1	64.2	61.2	62.0	63.0
2 or more	18.5	3.9	20.9	6.4
For Those With Sexual Partners, Routinely Use Condom				
Yes	37.5	35.6	56.2	29.1
Oral Intercourse In Last Year				
Yes	26.6	13.0	30.5	15.1
Anal Intercourse In Last Year				
Yes	3.3	4.3	6.7	2.5

Notes: * Number of sexual partners and oral intercourse significantly different by gender.
         **Number of sexual partners, condom use, oral intercosurse, and anal intercourse significantly different
         by age.

of the same sex. While these figures may be low compared to samples in large metropolitan areas, we believe they are an accurate reflection for the four counties studied, particularly since two of the counties are rural ones. Given some interesting and statistically significant differences in the sample by age and sex in terms of AIDS sexual practices, Table 2 shows these behaviors for age and sex groups. Almost double the percentage of women (35% versus 17%) reported no sexual partner in the past year. Similarly, men reported two or more sexual partners in the past year at a much higher rate (19%) than women (4%). Younger people under 30 were less likely to report no sexual partner (17 versus 30%) and more likely to report two or more (21 versus six percent) as compared to people 30 years of age and over. Oral intercourse was the only other sexual behavior in which differences by gender were statistically significant (27% for males versus 13% for females), although oral intercourse practices do not really change a person's risk of acquiring AIDS. Anal intercourse rates were generally quite low (under 5% for the total sample). Younger people were significantly more likely than those 30 and over to have routinely used a condom and to have engaged in oral or anal intercourse.

General knowledge levels about AIDS in the study were high and were typically higher on almost all items than national statistics from surveys in 1986 and 1987. Over 80 percent of people knew that a person can be infected with AIDS and not have the disease. Similarly, 87 percent knew you could not tell whether people had AIDS by simply looking at them. Almost everyone (94 percent) knew that the AIDS virus could be passed through sexual intercourse and that there was no cure for AIDS. In general, social and demographic characteristics were not associated with knowledge although levels of knowledge were in the rural counties were slightly lower. Due to the generally high levels of knowledge shown, we did not employ knowledge as a predictor of perceptions of risk. Sources of information were employed as a predictive variable for perceptions of risk of AIDS. Most people had many sources of information about AIDS. Out of nine possible sources of information, 17 percent of people reported three or more sources, 36 percent reported four or five, and 47 percent reported six or more.

Perceptions of Risk of AIDS and Comparisons with Other Diseases

Table 3 shows the means and standard deviations for the perceptions of risk of each of the eight health-problem items, including AIDS, divided by chances and seriousness. AIDS was very distinctive in terms of perceived chances. The mean for AIDS was only 1.5, between the lowest category of having no chance at all and the next category of extremely unlikely. Sixty-one percent of the sample perceived themselves to have no chance at all of contracting AIDS in the next five years. The estimated chances of developing other health problems all ranged from a mean of 3.3, the next lowest, for cancer up to a mean of 4.5 for sore throat. In general, the standard deviations indicated that the least dispersion on answers also occurred for the AIDS item, with the most for two of the more common and less serious health problems, sore throat and poison ivy.

The means on seriousness of various health problems also indicates how seriously AIDS is viewed (mean of 4.8 on a scale of 5; 94% perceive AIDS in the most serious category of 5), although the other two problems that are most immediately life-threatening, cancer (mean of 4.7) and heart problems (mean of 4.5), were also viewed fairly similarly in seriousness. The AIDS-seriousness item also had the smallest standard deviation (.7), followed by those for cancer (.8) and heart problems (.9). With the other problems, there is more variation on the seriousness scale, with sore throat and poison ivy being seen as not very serious (means of 1.7 and 1.8). High blood pressure and a serious car accident were also thought of as serious.

Explaining Differences in Perceptions of Risks

What types of factors help to explain variation in whether people perceive themselves to be at risk for AIDS and whether the disease is viewed as the most serious or some other, less serious category? We examined groups of demographic, health, and AIDS-behavior-related questions as independent variables which helped to predict variation in perceptions of risk of AIDS.

Table 3. Means and Standard Deviations for Perceptions of
AIDS and Other Diseases

	Mean	Standard Deviation
Chances to Contract (from 1 = no chance to 6 = extremely likely)		
AIDS	1.5	.8
High Blood Pressure	3.3	1.2
Sore Throat	4.5	1.3
Heart Problems	3.3	1.2
Cancer	3.3	1.2
Poison Oak or Ivy	3.6	1.3
Care Accident	3.8	.9
Cutting Yourself	3.9	1.0
Seriousness (from 1 = not severe to 5 = very severe)		
AIDS	4.8	.7
High Blood Pressure	4.1	1.0
Sore Throat	1.8	1.0
Heart Problems	4.5	.9
Cancer	4.7	.8
Poison Oak or Ivy	1.7	1.0
Care Accident	4.0	1.0
Cutting Yourself	2.8	1.1

Based on one-way analyses of variance for the continuous variables, we found that certain demographic and health variables were related to variations in perceptions of risk of AIDS. In general, the three health questions were only weakly associated with variation in perceived seriousness of AIDS. People who perceived their health as worse perceived their chances for acquiring AIDS as the lowest. Factors such as energy and worrying about a person's health were not related to perceptions of one's chances of acquiring AIDS or the perceived seriousness of AIDS. Some social and demographic factors were associated with perceived seriousness of AIDS. These included gender, urban/rural location, and income. Women perceived AIDS as even more serious than men. People in rural areas perceived AIDS as less serious. The lowest-income group perceived AIDS as less serious. There was a stronger correlation between social and demographic variables and perceived chances of developing AIDS. Younger people perceived their chances as higher, as did men, those living in urban areas and those with more education.

Three AIDS-related variables were also examined as independent variables: number of sexual partners, the total number of sources for AIDS information, and a measure of safer sexual practices in which no sexual partners or use

Table 4. Logistic Regression Analyses with Perceived chances of
AIDS as a Dependent Variable and Demographic, Health,
and AIDS Variables as Independent Variables

	Demographic Health Coefficients	AIDS Coefficients	Comprehensive Model Coefficients
Demographic Variables			
Education	.41**	—	.36**
Age	-.66**	—	-.58**
Race (2 = black)	-.01	—	.03
Gender (2 = female)	-.39	—	-.35
Marital Status (2 = not currently married)	.60**	—	.39
Income	-.08	—	
Urban/Rural (2 = rural)	-.32	—	-.54
Health Variables			
Self-Perceived	-.09	—	-.06
Worry	-.14	—	-.09
Energy	—	-.05	
AIDS Variables			
Number of Sexual Partners	—	.70**	.48
Number of Information Sources	—	-.12*	-.13*
Safe Practices (higher = safe practices)	—	.78***	.41*
Significance Level of Overall Model	< .0001	< .0001	< .001
$R^{2\dagger}$	.12	.06	.14

Notes: * $p < .05$.
       ** $p < .01$.
       † R^2 is a measure analogous to the usual adjusted R^2 for regression analysis, but is calculated differently because this is logistic regression.
       — Not in model.

of a condom were coded as safer and other practices as less safe. Number of sexual partners and number of sources of information were significant predictors of perceived chances of developing AIDS, with those with more sources of information less likely to perceive themselves as likely to develop AIDS. Those with more sexual partners perceived themselves at higher risk. The AIDS variables were not significant predictors of perceived seriousness of AIDS.

Univariate analysis tells only a partial story of factors which predict perceptions of risk. It is essential to go beyond univariate models because many of the predictors are themselves associated and thus the univariate models may tell only a partial or misleading story. After the examination of the distribution of the items related to perceived chances of developing AIDS and perceived

Table 5. Logistic Regression Analyses with Perceived Seriousness of
AIDS as a Dependent Variable and Demographic, Health,
and AIDS Variables as Independent Variables

	Demographic Health Coefficients	AIDS Coefficients	Comprehensive Model Coefficients
Demographic Variables			
Education	.13**	—	.15**
Age	-.67**	—	-.54*
Race (2 = black)	-.50	—	-.50
Gender (2 = female)	1.08	—	1.35**
Marital Status (2 = not currently married)	-.26	—	-.17
Income	.34	—	.32
Urban/Rural (2 = rural)	-.75	—	-.60*
Health Variables			
Self-Perceived	.19	—	.15
Worry	.36	—	.27
Energy	.18	—	.19
AIDS Variables			
Number of Sexual Partners	—	-.10	.18
Number of Information Sources	—	.02	.14
Safe Practices (higher = safe practices)	—	.34	.69
Significance Level of Overall Model	< .0001	NS	< .001
$R^{2\dagger}$	.12	.06	.14

Notes: * $p < .05$.
      ** $p < .01$.
      † R^2 is a measure analogous to the usual adjusted R^2 for regression analysis, but is calculated differently because this is logistic regression.
      — Not in model.

severity, we created three different dependent variables, each a zero-one variable was employed in a logistic-regression analysis. For likelihood, zero equals no chance at all and 1 equals some chance. For severity, one equals the most serious and zero equals all other categories of seriousness. The multiplicative variable is the product of likelihood times seriousness.

Tables 4, 5, and 6 present the multivariate logistic-regression models for the AIDS perceived risk questions as dependent variables. For perceived chances (likelihood), three demographic variables were significant predictors: age, education, and marital status. People with more education, younger people, and those not currently married all perceive themselves to have a greater chance of developing AIDs. Each of the AIDS variables is a significant predictor of

Table 6. Logistic Regression Analyses with Multiplicative Perceived Risk
of AIDS as a Dependent Variable and Demographic, Health,
and AIDS Variables as Independent Variables

	Demographic Health Coefficients	AIDS Coefficients	Comprehensive Model Coefficients
Demographic Variables			
Education	.41**	—	.36**
Age	-.65**	—	-.57**
Race (2 = black)	-.01	—	.002
Gender (2 = female)	-.30	—	-.22
Marital Status (2 = not currently married)	.60**	—	.33
Income	.02	—	-.06
Urban/Rural (2 = rural)	-.30	—	-.50*
Health Variables			
Self-Perceived	-.08	—	-.06
Worry	-.14	—	-.08
Energy	.03	—	.01
AIDS Variables			
Number of Sexual Partners	—	.72**	.37*
Number of Information Sources	—	-.12*	-.12
Safe Practices (higher = safe practices)	—	.67**	.57*
Significance Level of Overall Model	< .0001	< .0001	< .0001
$R^{2\dagger}$	.11	.05	.12

Notes: * $p < .05$.
    ** $p < .01$.
    † R^2 is a measure analogous to the usual adjusted R^2 for regression analysis, but is calculated differently because this is logistic regression.
    — Not in model.

perceived likelihood of developing AIDS. If a person has more sexual partners and practices fewer safe habits in the sexual area, perceived risk is higher. The more the information sources, the lower a person's perceives risk. In the comprehensive model, county (urban-rural location) is added in as an additional significant variable. Marital status and number of sexual partners are no longer significant predictors. In the comprehensive model, the analogous *R*-squared statistic is 14 percent.

Table 5 presents the logistic-regression analyses with perceived severity as the dependent variable. Only two demographic variables were significant predictors, age and gender. In the analysis with only the AIDS-related predictor, no AIDS variables were significant predictors of variability in perception of seriousness of AIDS. The model with only the AIDS variables explaining perception of seriousness was not statistically significant. In the comprehensive model, only the two demographic variables were significant and the comprehensive model does not predict significantly better than the model with demographic and health variables alone.

In the analyses with the multiplicative dependent variable, education, age, and marital status are the significant predictors among the demographic and health variables. In the analysis with AIDS-related variables, all three are significant predictors. In the comprehensive analysis, county becomes a significant predictor and marital status is less important. Only two of the AIDS variables remain as significant predictors. In none of the logistic-regression analyses are the health variables ever significant predictors. For the multiplicative perceived-risk variables, the same demographic factors are important as for perceived chances but there is some change in which AIDS variables are significant predictors.

In order to verify these analyses, stepwise logistic-regression analyses were applied to the three comprehensive models. With the exception of the variable of number of sexual partners becoming a significant predictor for perceived chances, the stepwise logistic-regression analyses confirmed the same predictors as important and found no other predictors significant.

CONCLUSIONS AND IMPLICATIONS

This study indicates that there is some, although fairly limited, variability in how people perceive both the seriousness and the likelihood of contracting AIDS. While people do perceive their own risks to be very, very low for acquiring AIDS, almost everyone sees it as extremely serious. In comparison to other diseases, heart disease and cancer were viewed as almost as serious. Thus certain notions of people's fear of disease may be relevant, and fears of AIDS may fit into more general societal fears of very serious diseases for which there are no cures or no simple and easy cures (Thomas 1987; Bean, Keller, Newburg, and Brown 1989).

Despite the limited variability in perceptions of severity of AIDS, adding the additional dimension of seriousness and a multiplicative function of likelihood times seriousness did add to the examination of perception of risk of AIDS. As treatment for AIDS improves and people with AIDS manage to live longer with the disease, the amount of variability in perceived seriousness may increase, making the use of both dimensions of perceived likelihood and severity even more useful in future research.

In the multivariate models, the better educated, the young, and the unmarried were likely to place their own chances of developing AIDS as higher than other groups, indicating that groups who would be likely to be at higher risk in a general population do share that perception. The importance of urban/ rural location (which is a significant predictor in the comprehensive models) has not been discussed in most other studies, although it appears that people living in rural areas perceive AIDS as less serious and less probable. The usefulness of demographic variables is in contrast to a Chicago study which did not find demographic variables to help explain perception of chances of contracting AIDS (Prohaska, Albrecht, Lekvy, Sugrue, and Kim 1990). AIDS-related measures alone did not help in explaining variation in perceptions of seriousness of AIDS but did in perception of chances of developing AIDS and the multiplicative function of overall perceived risk.

The way in which perceptions of AIDS in this sample were distinctive (both relative to other diseases and from some other AIDS-specific studies) was in people's low estimation of their own chances of acquiring AIDS in the next five years. The risk estimates in this study appear lower than those measured using different types of questions in some national studies and some studies in large metropolitan areas such as Chicago (Dawson and Thornberry 1988; Prohaska, Albrecht, Levy, Sugrue, and Kim 1990). Given the low rates of AIDS in South Carolina in 1989 and the low reported rates of risky behaviors related to AIDS, the perception of a person's own risk as being very, very low may be accurate. One important conclusion for public-health efforts in the future is that as long as many people view themselves as having no real probability of contracting AIDS (over 60% of the people in this study estimated that they had no chance of contracting AIDS in the next five years), educational efforts focused on teaching people safe sexual practices and other ways to protect themselves from AIDS will probably have no impact on this large group of people. If one perceives oneself as at no risk of contracting AIDS, then messages about needed behavior changes will probably not receive any attention, since the interpretation is that they are relevant only for those other people (with some risk) not oneself who is estimated to be at no risk. Yet recent national data indicate that AIDS is increasing in rural areas and some part of the country where rates were previously quite low. For future educational campaigns to impact a population such as that in South Carolina or other states with low rates and rural areas, it may first be necessary to convince people that they have *any* chance of contracting the disease. This may need to be the focus of mass media campaigns particularly, since messages of how to change behavior will not have an impact on people who see themselves at no risk.

REFERENCES

Albrecht, G.L., J.A. Levy, N. M. Sugrue, T.R. Prohaska, and D.G. Ostrow. 1989. "Who Hasn't Heard About AIDS?" *AIDS Education and Prevention* 1: 261-267.
Allard, R. 1989. "Beliefs About AIDS Determinants of Preventive Practices and of Support For Coercive Measures." *American Journal of Public Health* 79: 448-452.

Bean, J., L. Keller, C. Newburg, and M. Brown. 1989. "Methods for the Reduction of AIDS Social Anxiety and Social Stigma." *AIDS Education and Prevention* 1: 194-221.

Becker, M.H. 1974. "The Health Belief Model and Sick Role Behavior." *Health Education Monographs* 2: 409-420.

Becker, M.H. and N.K. Janz. 1987. "On the Effectiveness and Utility of Health Hazard/Health Risk Appraisal in Clinical and Nonclinical Settings." *Health Services Research* 22: 537-551.

Becker, M.H. and J.G. Joseph. 1988. "AIDS and Behavioral Change to Reduce Risk: A Review." *American Journal of Public Health* 78: 394-410.

Becker, D. and D. Levine. 1987. "Risk Perception, Knowledge, and Lifestyles in Siblings of People With Premature Coronary Disease." *American Journal of Preventive Medicine* 3: 45-50.

Belloc, N.B., L. Breslow, and J.R. Hochstim. 1971. "Measures of Physical Health In a General Population Survey." *American Journal of Epidemiology* 93: 328-336.

Berkman, L.F. and L. Breslow. 1983. *Health and Ways of Living: The Alameda County Study.* New York: Oxford University Press.

Cleary, P.D., T.F. Rogers, E. Singer, J. Avorn, N. Van Devanter, S. Perry, and J. Pindyck. 1986. "Health Education About AIDS Among Seropositive Blood Donors." *Health Education Quarterly* 13: 317-329.

Dawson, D. National Center For Health Statistics. 1990. *AIDS Knowledge and Attitudes for January-March, 1990.* Advance Data from Vital and Health Statistics No. 193. DHHS Pub. No (PHS) 90-1250. Hyattesville, Md: Public Health Service.

Dawson, D. and M. Hardy. National Center for Health Statistics. 1989. *AIDS Knowledge and Attitudes of Black Americans. Provisional Data from the National Health Survey.* Advance Data from Vital and Health Statistics No. 165. DHHS Pub. No. (PHS) 89-1250. Hyattesville, MD: Public Health Service.

Dawson D. and O. Thornberry. National Centre For Health Statistics. 1988. *Aids Knowledge and Attitudes for December, 1987. Provisional Data From the National Health Interview Survey.* Advance Data From Vital and Health Statistics No. 165. DHHS Pub. No (PHS) 89-1250. Hyattesville, MD: Public Health Service.

DiClimente, R., C. Boyer, and E. Morales. 1988. "Minorities and AIDS: Knowledge, Attitudes, and Misconceptions Among Black and Latino Adolescents." *American Journal of Public Health* 78: 55-57.

DiClimente, R.J., J. Zorn, and L. Temoshok. 1986. "Adolescents and AIDS: A Survey of Knowledge, Attitudes and Beliefs About AIDS in San Francisco." *American Journal of Public Health* 76: 1443-1445.

Douglas, M. 1985. *Risk Acceptability According to the Social Sciences.* New York: Russell Sage.

Emmons, C.A., J.G. Joseph, R.C. Kessler, C.B. Wortman, S.B. Montgomery, and D.G. Ostrow. 1986. "Psychosocial Predictors of Reported Behavior Change in Homosexual Men At Risk For AIDS." *Health Education Quarterly* 13: 331-345.

Fischoff, B., P. Slovic, and S. Lichenstein. 1978. "How Safe is Safe Enough? A Psychometric Study of Attitudes Toward Technological Risks and Benefits." *Policy Sciences* 9: 127-152.

Frey, J.H. 1983. *Survey Research By Telephone.* Beverly Hills, CA Sage.

Glik, D., J. Kronenfeld, and K. Jackson. Forthcoming. "Predictors of Risk Perceptions of Childhood Injury Among Parents of Preschoolers." *Health Education Quarterly.*

Groves, R.M. 1989. *Survey Error and Total Cost.* New York: Wiley.

Groves, R.M. and R.L. Kahn. 1979. *Survey By Telephone: A National Comparison With Personal Interview.* New York: Academic Press.

Janz, N.K. and M.H. Becker. 1984. "The Health Belief Model: A Decade Later." *Health Education Quarterly* 11: 1-47.

Joseph, J.G., S.B. Montgomery, C.A. Emmons, R.C. Kessler, D.G. Ostrow, C.B. Wortman, K. O'Brien, M. Eller, and S. Eshleman. 1987. Magnitudes and Determinants of Behavioral

Risks to Health: Longitudinal Analyses of a Cohort At Risk for AIDS." *Psychological Health* 1: 73-96.

Kahneman, D. and A. Tversky. 1979a. "Subjective Probabilities: A Judgment of Representativeness." *Cognitive Psychology* 3: 430-455.

_____. 1979b. "Prospect Theory: An Analysis of Decision Under Risk." *Econometrica* 47: 263-291.

_____. 1982. *Judgment Under Uncertainty: Heuristics and Biases.* New York: Cambridge University Press.

Koopman, C., J. Rotheram-Borus, R. Henderson, J. Bradley, and J. Hunter. 1990. "Assessment of Knowledge About AIDS and Beliefs About AIDS Prevention Among Adolescents." *AIDS Education and Prevention* 2: 58-70.

Kronenfeld, J.J. and D.C. Glik. 1990. "Perception of Risk: Applicability in Medical Sociological Research." Pp. 307-344 in *Research in the Sociology of Health Care,* Vol. 9. edited by D. Wertz. Greenwich, CT: JAI Press.

Marin, G. 1989. "AIDS Prevention Among Hispanics: Needs, Risk Behaviors, and Cultural Values." *Public Health Reports* 104: 411-415.

McCusker, J., J. Zapka, A. Stoddard, and K. Mayer. 1989. Responses to the AIDS Epidemic Among Homosexually Active Men: Factors Associated with Preventive Behavior." *Patient Education and Counseling* 13: 15-30.

McKusick, L, W. Horstman, and T.J. Coates. 1985. "AIDS and Sexual Behavior Reported By Gay Men In San Francisco." *American Journal of Public Health* 75: 493-496.

Nelkin, D. 1989. "Communicating Technological Risk: The Social Construction of Risk Perception" *Annual Review of Public Health* 10: 95-113.

Neubauer, B.J. 1989. "Risk-Taking, Responsibility For Health and Attitudes Toward Avoiding AIDS." *Psychological Reports* 64: 1255-1260.

Niknian, M., S. McKinlay, W. Rakowski, R. Carleton. 1989. "A Comparison of Perceived and Objective CVD Risk in a General Population." *American Journal of Public Health* 79:1653-1654.

Nisbett, R. and L. Ross. 1980. *Human Inference: Strategies and Shortcomings of Social Judgment.* Englewood Cliffs, NJ: Prentice-Hall.

Prohaska, T.R., G. Albrecht, J. Levy, N. Sugrue, and J. Kim. 1990. "Determinants of Self-Perceived Risk for AIDS." *Journal of Health and Social Behavior* 31: 384-394.

Singer, E., T.F. Roger, M. Corcoran. 1987. "The Polls—A Report." *Public Opinion Quarterly* 51: 580-595.

Slovic, P. 1987. "Perception of Risk." *Science* 236: 280-285.

Slovic, P., B. Fischoff, and S. Lichenstein. 1978. "Accident Probabilities and Seat Belt Usage: A Psychological Perspective." *Accident Analysis and Prevention* 10: 281-285.

_____. 1977. "Behavioral Decision Theory." *Annual Review of Psychology* 28: 1-39.

Szasz, A. 1988. "Risk Perception Research and Modern Social Theory." Paper presented at the American Sociological Association Annual Meeting, Atlanta, GA.

Stall, R., L. McKusick, J. Wiley, T.J. Coates, and D.G. Ostrow. 1986. "Alcohol and Drug Use During Sexual Activity and Compliance With Safe Sex Guideline for AIDS: The AIDS Behavioral Research Project." *Health Education Quarterly* 13: 359-371.

Taylor-Nicholson, M., M. Wang, and D. Adame. 1989. "Impact of AIDS Education on Adolescent Knowledge, Attitudes and Perceived Susceptibility." *Health Values* 13: 3-7.

Thompson, L.M. 1987. "Dealing With AIDS and Fear: Would You Accept Cookies From an AIDS Patient?" *Southern Medical Journal* 80: 228-232.

Thompson, P. 1990. "Risk Objectivism and Risk Subjectivism: When Are Risks Real?" *Issues in Health and Safety* 1: 3-22.

Tversky, A. and D. Kahneman. 1974. "Judgment Under Uncertainty: Heuristics and Biases." *Science* 185: 1124-1131.

Weinstein, N.D. 1980. "Unrealistic Optimism About Future Life Events." *Journal of Personality and Social Psychology* 39: 806-820.

_____. 1982. "Unrealistic Optimism About Susceptibility to Health Problems." *Journal of Behavioral Medicine* 5: 441-460.

_____, ed. 1987. *Taking Care.* Cambridge, England: Cambridge University Press.

Wildavsky, A. 1982. *Risk and Culture.* Berkeley: University of California Press.

Windle, M. 1989. "High-Risk Behaviors for AIDS Among Heterosexual Alcoholics: A Pilot Study." *Journal of Studies on Alcohol* 50: 503-507.

FROM EPIDEMIC TO MODERN ILLNESS:
THE SOCIAL CONSTRUCTION OF AIDS IN FRANCE

Claudine Herzlich and Janine Pierret

ABSTRACT

The meanings and metaphors attached to AIDS have paralleled advances in medicine. Through naming processes and statistics, the press made news about this specialized subject into a general topic polarizing social relations. Explained in terms of an epidemic, a notion with inappropriate connotations from the past, the "AIDS social phenomenon" raises ethical issues and exposes the inadequacy of the health system, the hesitancy of political decision making, and the limits of medicine. Its autonomy limited, the medical profession has had to cooperate with other actors, in particular, activist AIDS organizations. Given the medical sciences' relative impotence as therapy lags behind research, prevention work and the modification of behaviors have assumed importance, and public authorities have turned toward the social sciences. The latter have resorted to history, since behavior patterns reach back to bygone afflictions. AIDS-related research may decompartmentalize the sociology of illness in France and broaden its perspectives.

The Social and Behavioral Aspects of AIDS.
Advances in Medical Sociology, Volume 3, pages 59-76.

INTRODUCTION

AIDS has made us the unwilling spectators of a seldom occurring event: the outbreak of a new illness, its sudden irruption into public life and collective consciousness. During every past epoch, one or more diseases prevailed in the collective imagination and had unsettling effects on the social order. Campaigns against them, as well as the treatment of casualties, mobilized society's human and financial resources. Symbolically, such diseases were a prevalent way of "embodying" collective and individual misfortunes. They cried out for an explanation to tell the truth about both the sick body and world order. They starkly exposed the relations between biological, political, and social realities.

These preliminary comments lead us to raise questions about how our own society has, in a very short time, "constructed this new reality" (Berger and Luckmann 1966). First, how has AIDS become a social phenomenon affecting the whole society, crystallizing strong emotions, and polarizing social relations? Second, what does the medical care for persons with AIDS (henceforth, PWAs) in France teach us about the relations between medicine, science, politics, public opinion, and these persons? After trying to answer these questions, we conclude with a few comments about the impact of AIDS on the social sciences, in particular sociology.

THE PRESS'S ROLE IN RESUSCITATING BYGONE CONCEPTIONS OF DISEASE

This new illness makes us hark back to a nearly forgotten theme: disease as punishment and epidemics as a scourging of society. By combining sociological and historical approaches, Herzlich and Pierret (1987) have shown how the diseases and the sick of the past have become the illnesses and patients of today. Illness is considered, in all current analyses of illness, including medical sociology, to be a form that an individual life's may take. To be chronically ill, today's prevalent type of illness, refers to more than a biological state. In the past, the contagiousness, or infectiousness, of a disease state turned a biological phenomenon into a social reality. Nowadays, to be ill generally refers to a status and implies the reception of health care. In other words, the person enters into a relationship with a major institution: medicine. People who are ill may live for years while keeping up social activities and without representing a threat to those around them.

Illness increasingly corresponds to an identity to be assumed, won, and imposed on others. The relationship with the institution of medicine is one way, among others, of forming this identity. Illness as a way of life and the patient as a social actor are very different from what happened over previous centuries during epidemics. The latter were social phenomena embodying absolute evil, or misfortune. Paradoxically, they were also "diseases without patients" since they mainly corresponded to ways of dying. From Boccaccio to Pepys and Chateaubriand, from Thucydides to Manzoni and Defoe, many accounts have been written about epidemics. When reading them, what strikes us most is the repetitiveness. All of them point to: the number of victims; the suddenness of death; the lack of efficacious means for stopping the epidemic; behaviors such as panic, flight, and debauchery; and the breakdown of social order. In the early 1980s, a new pathology arose and the ancient label "epidemic" was soon stuck onto it. The intensity of reactions proves the relevance of distinguishing between yesterday's and today's illnesses. This new "epidemic" was a shock: it should not have happened; it was inconceivable nowadays; everything would change as a result. We would like to analyze how the bygone theme of an epidemic has been linked to the modern notion of illness. How has AIDS been used to make this linkage in collective discourses and representations as well as in facts and practices?[1]

This new "AIDS reality" has been constructed through rapid advances made in biology and epidemiology since, in the United States in 1980-1981, the first cases were signaled of young men, usually homosexuals, who were suffering from various symptoms and whose immune systems had broken down. The mass media instantly reported live on this new illness. The press, in particular, made AIDS come into being for the general public. The results of the recent surveys on Knowledge, Attitudes, Beliefs, and Practices carried out under the auspices of the World Health Organization (WHO) in more than 60 countries in Europe, the Americas, and Africa reveal that, in every country and regardless of the number of AIDS cases there, the population was always first informed through the media. In the early 1980s, when this new illness affected barely more than a few hundred persons dispersed in various places, AIDS had already become, the West at least, something everybody knew about and commented on. According to Veron (1981, pp. 7-8):

> Social events are not objects that exist already made somewhere in reality and that the media inform us about—about their properties and avatars—subsequently and more or less accurately. They only exist inasmuch as the media shape them.

AIDS was shaped in two ways as a social event. First, the press announced a new pathology, gradually described it, and in particular, turned news about it from being a specialized, scientific, or medical subject into a topic of general concern. The phrase "AIDS social phenomenon," as French journalists put it, reveals how the mass media identified and classified the events they were reporting. Second, AIDS became a social phenomenon as the press circulated news about it among social groups that would gradually feel concerned and as relations polarized. It thus became a social issue on which political parties took positions and over which they clashed. Public opinion, an imprecise category that exists, first of all, in the idea one has of it, has always been present in the AIDS phenomenon.[2]

AN INEXPLICABLE ACCIDENT

We can point out the phases in the construction of this social phenomenon. Six months went by before French dailies followed up on articles in the internationally renowned *New England Journal of Medicine* about a "mysterious" illness observed in the United States during the spring of 1981. On January 6, 1982, *Libération* inquired about this "mysterious cancer among American homosexuals" (see Conan 1982) and *Le Quotidien de Paris,* about a "strange illness affecting homosexuals." On January 27, *Le Monde* devoted its medicine section to this new illness under the heading "Why Cancers?" (see Escoffier-Mambiotte 1982). This serious, mysterious disease had been detected through routine data collection by the Center for Disease Control (CDC) at Atlanta in the United States. The first hypotheses about immune deficiency were based on inferences, as the French public learned thanks to *Le Figaro's* first article which, in March 1983, stated that the CDC had observed an abnormal consumption of lomidine, a drug used for treating pneumoncystis, one of the AIDS-related opportunistic infections (see Vigy 1983).

According to Goody (1977), various techniques, simple in principle, for tallying, visualizing, and recording (tables, lists, and formulas) have been especially helpful in the evolution of a scientific mentality. Since the facts handled by science are not immediately "visible," it is necessary to develop means for measuring and recording results, according to Latour (1985), so as to perceive basic trends, whether in the French economy or the outbreak of a disease. In the case of AIDS, it has been amazing to observe the effectiveness, and speed, of recording procedures. Epidemiological surveillance signaled a new phenomenon, made it "visible," and immediately sought data for corroborating this reality. The CDC soon sized up the situation: the number and types of affected persons as well as of infectious agents and, especially, major immunodeficiency.

In 1981 and 1982, very few persons actually "saw" this new illness. As a March 1982 article in *La Recherche* pointed out, there were "nearly more" New York and Californian doctors interested in it than there were casualties. In fact, there were few of either. For a long time, the French press stayed silent. But once the first articles came out, those who saw what was happening (the first doctors in contact with the first AIDS patients) pointed out how serious this new illness was. The first journalists to cover this new story did not fail to mention this while citing names (Dr. Leibowitch at Raymond Poincaré Hospital and Dr. Rozenbaum at Claude Bernard Hospital). Articles even went so far as to comment on the "suddenness with which the disease appeared"

(Sauclières 1982, p. 393) and describe it as a mystery neither understandable nor explicable with current knowledge.

From the outset, the French press presented the new illness as a medical mystery, in this respect similar to the American Legion disease or to the inexplicable deaths in Spain that had followed the ingestion of adulterated olive oil. There was a tone of uncertainty, ignorance, or even stupefaction in these articles, which saw this inexplicable accident interrupting the ordinary course of life, perhaps—although no one was yet sure—for a long time. In May 1983, when the first solid findings were made, a consensus emerged among scientists, and the phenomenon was "stabilized" for the first time. Until then, press articles had popularized hypotheses formulated in medical circles and scientific journals. Doctors and researchers were the sources, whether mentioned or not. However, these sources turned out not to know very much. The variety of hypotheses strengthened the feeling that nothing was known for sure. Although some dailies had, from the start, mentioned eventual public-health issues, the new illness was not yet a social phenomenon whose cultural, social, or ethical aspects would provoke interpretations.

THE MAKING OF A SOCIAL PHENOMENON

During the first half of 1983, the new illness gradually ceased being a medical mystery and became a well identified, though still unexplained, biological object. This took place through a naming process. Besides naming the new phenomenon, this process brought into focus images of the illness and also of group conflicts. The same questions ("Who names it?" and "What is being named?") would crop up again, a few years later, when the virus was to be named. Until July 1983, all labels stuck onto the illness referred to homosexuals, the most affected group: "homosexuals' pneumonia," "homosexual cancer," "gay cancer," "syndrome of homosexuals," or "gay syndrome." Several articles, even as they used these names, pointed out their inaccuracy. As early as the summer of 1982, the press had reported that homosexuals were not the only group concerned since the illness also struck Haitians, drug-users, and even children. Likewise, it was pointed out that this new illness was not a kind of cancer. Despite efforts to be objective and accurate, the immediately forceful association in symbolic and social terms was winning out.

In March 1983, several French dailies started using the English medical abbreviation, AIDS, which would be translated a few months later as *SIDA* (*syndrome d'immuno-déficience acquise*). Two aspects of this naming process should be emphasized. First, the English term was translated into French, whereas the term "AIDS" was adopted in many other languages. In 1983, a quarrel broke out between the research teams headed by Professor Gallo of NIH (United States) and Professor Montagnier of Institut Pasteur (France); and it was necessary to adopt a definite name in French for the new illness. Second, the adoption of a scientific name was an attempt to remain neutral, as an article in *Le Figaro* on March 22, 1983 stated, "The current names are less telling, but they have the advantage of corresponding to biological and medical reality" (see Vigy 1983). The new name diffused slowly: from March to July 1983, all articles (about 30, several on front pages) added it onto "homosexual syndrome" or "gay cancer." It would eventually be widely adopted and written in small letters *(sida)*. This language neutrality would soon be broken, as negative connotations were loaded onto the new name. AIDS—and this was the issue in its construction as a social phenomenon—would come to symbolize whatever was threatening or shameful, and its victims would become targets of accusations and discrimination. AIDS became a metaphor for what was wrong not just with the body. In December 1986, a far-right journalist, L. Pauwels in *Le Figaro,* would refer to modern society as being corrupt and degenerate, as having "mental AIDS."

Another process—statistical—popularized AIDS, this time as an epidemiological reality. Statistics about AIDS "victims" were run in newspapers. As early as February 1982, *Libération* summed up 159 cases in the United States in November 1981 plus 57 new cases during the following two months, making a total of 216, including 88 deaths. The first two AIDS articles in 1982 (on January 6) mentioned a case in France. In February, five cases were tallied, and some doctors began trying to set up procedures for keeping track. On February 6, *Libération* wrote, "A few doctors motivated by their specialties have improvised an informal coordination center for circulating initial information." Thereafter, the French press would regularly publish statistics from the CDC, WHO, and Ministry of Health.

AIDS was spreading fast—the French dailies harped on this idea, and the association was inevitably made with an epidemic. Although the absolute number of persons affected was very small and would stay so for some time, statistics were used not only to give an idea about the spread of the disease but also to show that what had, until then, been deemed a temporary accident was, in fact, an irreversible, nonrandom phenomenon. In other words, the accidental was becoming permanent. New stories told about a risky, hard-to-control situation and continually mixed up current statistics with predictions (or expectations) about the disease's potentially limitless extension. The time scale shifted: there was an emergency. To confront the ever worsening danger, "something had to be done."

Given this biological menace, the only intelligible explanatory model was an epidemic. This model would precipitate other themes related to the moral and cultural aspects of sickness. In particular, the ancient idea of disease as punishment would weigh heavily on certain groups. Before AIDS, the themes of blood, sex, guilt, and punishment had already been brought together to talk about another sexually transmitted disease, genital herpes. In the early 1980s, the French press had run articles about the "herpes psychosis" that, associated with sex, had also broken out in the United States. There was already talk about an epidemic, a term already associated with notions of contagion, panic, and divine punishment. The press mentioned that, in American society, some persons with herpes had suffered from discrimination and that the first signs of a "moralization of sexual practices" could be seen. Genital herpes foreshadowed AIDS. It fueled heated debates and set off reactions, especially in the United States. But in France, too, a pattern of symbols had formed that would soon be updated, with an unprecedented emotional impact, for AIDS.

MORAL DISCOURSES AND ADVANCES IN KNOWLEDGE

The meaning attributed to this unknown illness, and the metaphors attached to it, changed in line with advances in medical knowledge. The first epidemiological data became available in April 1982, and the French dailies started using the phrase "risk factor" when talking about homosexuals. In the spring of 1983, articles were run about the first results of research on the AIDS virus. For the first time too, journalists reported about AIDS' impact on American "homosexual communities."

Taken from probability and referring to a statistical correlation, the concept of risk as in risk group was too often used to refer to a direct causal link between AIDS and homosexuality. The concept of a biological risk was thus bound up with "homosexual life-styles" even though studies, in particular Pollak's (1988), have clearly shown that "homosexual life-style" and "homosexual community," rather than designating a homogeneous reality, cover quite different practices, senses of identity, and group memberships.

This ambiguous mixture of risk and causality overlapped with two ideas about how AIDS was "transmitted." The idea that the disease was transmitted mostly among homosexuals carried the meaning that it was a curse upon the guilty. And the idea that AIDS was out of control and would spread everywhere meant that it was a catastrophe that would kill more and more people. Were homosexuals victims of AIDS? Were they "guilty" of having or spreading it? Moralistic replies were made about the origin of the curse and, especially, about the responsibility for a catastrophe that affects others than oneself. This discourse resuscitated the ancient theme of the "flawed body" (Herzlich and Pierret 1987, ch. 9): in late nineteenth-century France, the belief was rife that syphilis resulted from a "fault" or "crime" committed against the body, lineage, or race. AIDS thus served to link a traditional conception of illness with a scientific concept borrowed from epidemiology, a discipline of which most of the population had never heard.

By the summer of 1983 (as had happened during the plague), this new illness provided the opportunity for projecting negative images onto "others" (homosexuals, drug-users, Americans, Haitians, and, later, Africans) and proclaiming them guilty. Accusations, denials, and guilt prevailed in news

about AIDS. These images, as emotionally laden as they were, were also used
to cognitive ends. Their variety would help journalists understand AIDS and
make projections about its development. Apprehension was thus fueled about
the spread of the disease—both its geographical extension and the increasing
number of casualties. After the United States, countries in Europe and then
Africa were being added to the list. And what about Eastern Europe and Asia
which seemed to have been spared?

Although "others" were assigned the lead role as victims, whether guilty or
not, the French press presented them in other roles too. One was as rival during
the French-American "scientific war" that, for several months, took place
between two research teams, each claiming to have discovered the AIDS virus.
The "other" also served as a positive model, when journalists reported on AIDS
among American homosexuals and the measures being taken against this new
disease. Readers were thus led to imagine the future and shown how to react.
However, the discourses about "others" were often discourses attributed to
others—when speakers did not assume responsibility for them. French
journalists, for example, M. Szafran in *Le Matin* on June 21, 1983, attributed
interpretations of AIDS as a divine punishment to the "Puritan Anglo-Saxon
mentality," "Reaganism," and the "moral order" spreading over the United
States in the early 1980s. Regardless of personal positions, everybody was
affected by this discourse. A meaning was being built up around AIDS and
forced upon everyone, even if some wanted to deny it. This meaning had to
do with a concrete threat that concerned everybody, not just homosexuals—
a threat against late twentieth-century values and culture. The French press
thus began writing about the "AIDS effect" and the "AIDS social
phenomenon."

The same reactions occurred during the summer of 1985 when, in a chain
reaction from the United States to European countries, panic broke out in
certain settings. Once again, a scientific breakthrough set off emotional
reactions and a process of stigmatization. This breakthrough was the test for
detecting the presence of the AIDS virus in the human body. People who where
HIV positive would, initially, be called healthy carriers (*porteurs sains*). News
about this new technique brought to mind a danger that was all the more deadly
because it was hidden: the theme of contagion reappeared, as did the idea that
AIDS could potentially spread throughout society and over the world. Violent
reactions were set off when healthy carriers, sometimes a single person were
discovered in certain settings (the reactions of prison guards toward HIV-
positive inmates or of parents with children in a school attended by a HIV-
positive child). When reporting these stories, the press's position and language
were ambiguous. By addressing minorities "at risk" as well as the general public,
by trying to "dedramatize" while reporting such events and often criticizing
extreme reactions, newspapers were placed in a double bind: they seemed to
be "denying what they affirmed and affirming what they denied" (Pollak, Dab,

and Moatti 1989, p. 129), namely the imminence of a catastrophe and the guilt of "risk groups." During the summer of 1985, AIDS became a daily topic in the papers. The press tried to provide news so as to quell emotions. Nonetheless, fear seemed to be growing as news spread.

A NEW ACTOR: THE HIV-POSITIVE

The test for the presence of the AIDS virus brought into being a new group, the HIV-positive (*séropositif*). Persons in this group, although they are not sick, have had to face up to and manage a complicated, uncertain, suspicion-ridden situation. Transmitted by bodily substances, this new illness has resuscitated the fear of contagion. Everybody is a danger for everybody else. This fear is all the stronger given that AIDS associates sexuality with death and fells young people of reproductive age.

The "contaminated" have to manage everyday life despite uncertainty and surveillance (Weitz 1989). A question has gradually loomed over their lives: when and how will they fall sick? There are no answers, but the menace exists. It thus becomes important to take precautions especially, and sometimes exclusively, against contracting AIDS during sexual intercourse. Fears of infecting others and reinfecting oneself have led to changes in sexual behaviors, sometimes as radical as abstinence. To manage their lives, the HIV-positive have changed health habits by, for example, getting enough sleep, decreasing the consumption of alcoholic beverages, or eating "natural," balanced meals. (Few have given up smoking however.) These changes bring to mind the "duty to be healthy" (Herzlich and Pierret 1987, ch. 12) but in a context of defense against AIDS. Managing uncertainty and the "flawed body" call for paying close, almost daily, attention to one's body and watching for the smallest signs.

The shift from HIV-positive to PWA occurs when biological parameters are kept under regular surveillance by medical practitioners. The relationship to medicine, to medical care and techniques, objectifies the illness and turns those who refuse to recognize they are sick into patients. Close bonds often form between PWAs and health professionals, bonds all the stronger insofar as they form between age-mates. In fact, nearly all doctors who followed up on the first PWAs or HIV-positive persons were young too. Relations between doctors and PWAs have often been intensely emotional. (This is not the first time this has happened; cf. Fox's [1959] notion of a red-carpet treatment.) In France, the cultural and generational similarities between those in need of care and those providing care have helped them strive together against disease and death.

The hardest problem to manage is secrecy. Should others be told that someone is HIV-positive? If so, who should be told, and when? Although positions on this question are not very clear-cut, the answers, though diverse, have a single objective: to avoid discrimination and "marginalization." PWAs and HIV-positive people often feel ashamed of their sick, dangerous bodies. Hence, it is necessary to struggle against and reject feelings of shame for being stricken with an illness that reveals one's way of life to others. For this reason, AIDS is not just an illness. Certain activists have committed themselves to this struggle by refusing to be ashamed of being sick. In a February 1984 article in *Le Monde*, Blaudin de Thé, a cancerologist returning from the United States, voiced these feelings when he emphasized the importance of this activism since PWAs "become, in a way, 'pariahs,' all of them deeply affected in their moral, social and physical selves." In 1991, negative attitudes toward PWAs and HIV-positive people persist despite television campaigns and interviews with the intent of making these groups visible. The cleavage still exists between "innocent victims" (hemophiliacs and children) and the "others." The improved visibility of AIDS has had ambivalent effects.

A MODERN EPIDEMIC?

Bourdelais (1989), a historian, is right when he affirms that the closest similarity between AIDS today and the epidemics of yesterday lies in individual and collective reactions: behaviors, indeed, persist on a long-term scale. The foregoing analysis has shed light on how ideas and images from the past have been resuscitated. When making a social and medical comparison between AIDS and past epidemics, we are forced to recognize dissimilarities. True, AIDS contradicts our belief that the era of infectious diseases is over. Even though biologists think that other, in particular viral, infections may break out, there are many dissimilarities between AIDS and past epidemics.

First, mortality rates in the total population differ. In the 14th century, the Black Death wiped out a quarter of Western Europe's population within a few months (Herzlich and Pierret 1987; Delumeau and Lequin 1987). Even in the nineteenth century, the mortality rate shot up because of cholera (Bourdelais and Raulot 1987). So far, AIDS has caused nothing of similar in developed nations. From 1982 to March 31, 1991, the total number of cases (including deaths) in France was 14,449. In the fall of 1990, an official report (Brunet et al. 1990), while exposing the difficulty of obtaining accurate statistics, estimated that from 100 to 200 thousand Frenchpersons have been infected by the HIV virus and risk contracting full-blown AIDS. These estimates, though impressive, do not meet the dire predictions made between 1983 and 1985. Foretelling the future is even harder. Experts think that the infection rate has decreased among homosexuals but stayed the same, or even increased, among intravenous drug-users (henceforth IVDUs), as well as heterosexual men and women. Although AIDS is less deadly for the general population than epidemics used to be, infected individuals run more risks of dying—they had a better chance of surviving the bubonic plague! In the nineteenth century, one out of two persons sick with cholera recovered (Bourdelais and Raulot 1987).

Another difference between AIDS and past epidemics is the speed. The latter struck suddenly, and the infected died within a few days. In contrast, AIDS slowly creeps up, and the incubation period is now thought to last from seven to 12 years. This has ambiguous effects on groups and individuals as they apprehend the illness: they have time to be overcome by anxiety but also to prepare for, even forestall, being sick. For this reason, and given the major way AIDS is transmitted, the closest similarity is not with the plague, as has usually been suggested, but with syphilis.

Finally, there is, it should be pointed out, not one but several AIDS "epidemics." This holds biologically as well as epidemiologically. According to Grmek (1989) and Mann, the former director of WHO's AIDS program, (Mann, Chin, Piot, and Quinn 1988) various viruses are involved, and AIDS is spread in a variety of ways. Rapid changes have put an end to simplistic, initial comparisons. In fact, HIV-positive people differ considerably from region to region (IVDUs and homosexuals in the United States and Western Europe, heterosexuals in Africa). However, the AIDS "epidemics"—if this term is to be used—also differ as a function of cultural and economic contexts, of the financial, social, and medical resources available, and, therefore, of the provision of health care. In this sense, AIDS is, indeed, an illness of our times since it starkly highlights the inequality between nations (between the North and South, between Western lands and Africa) as they fight against disease. The necessary medical and economic cooperation seems to be still wanting. As Rozenberg (1989, p. 11) has stated:

> AIDS might well be described as modern and even postmodern in its relationship to scientific medicine and institutional structures. AIDS is postmodern in the self-conscious, reflexive and bureaucratically structured detachment with which we regard it.

THE STATE AND MEDICINE FACING A MODERN EPIDEMIC

It is not easy to briefly analyze collective responses in France to AIDS, nor to interpret the characteristics of this illness of our times. It is easy to declare, from the start, that AIDS has exposed: the inadequacy of the health care system, the slowness and hesitancy of political decision-making processes[3], the limits of medicine and of medical research, and complicating ethical factors. Though at the origin of new problems, AIDS has more often brought to light difficulties that had previously been eluded. Paradoxically, it has also served, nationally and internationally, as the basis for an unprecedented mobilization of people and resources against an illness; and it has displayed our societies' capacity for responding.

AIDS broke into French politics in 1985, when the state (as during the centuries of epidemics—on a long-term scale) became concerned about protecting the population. Because AIDS was spread through contaminated blood, the problem of routinely testing blood donors led, in the summer, to a national strategy. Prime Minister Fabius himself intervened, and the government decided on August 1 to routinely test blood donors. This proved that AIDS was no longer the private problem of the ill or the professional problem of doctors. It had become an issue for which the government had to assume responsibility and which politicians would not fail to address. The time when this occurred was meaningful: in the summer of 1985, three-and-a-half years after the detection of the first cases in France. In the meantime, public opinion had become aware of AIDS and was worrying about the disease spreading widely. Two years later, Prime Minister Chirac would negotiate an agreement with the United States for recognizing the joint discovery of the AIDS virus by Gallo and Montagnier. In 1987, centers opened for anonymous HIV-testing free of charge. In early 1989, the government set up institutions for AIDS research, prevention work, and discussion of ethical problems, respectively: the National Agency of AIDS Research (*Agence Nationale de Recherche sur le Sida*), the French Agency for Campaigns against AIDS (*Agence Française de Lutte contre le Sida*), and the National AIDS Council (*Conseil National du Sida*).

From the start, doctors had a central position in managing this new illness. Enormous medical and scientific investments turned AIDS into the paradigm of modern illness. Doctors, once the first cases had been detected, became active and organized, in France as in the United States. Hospital services in Paris quickly made special efforts to handle the first cases. Research started; the Institut Pasteur published findings about the virus in the spring of 1983. Doctors, notedly the psychiatrist Didier Seux, innovated social changes in patient care. During the congress of the Gay Doctors' Association (*Association des Médecins Gays*) in the spring of 1982, the first information was diffused toward French homosexuals—in the midst of controversy.

The medical profession's key position, as well as its various roles, was evidence that it had become the prototype of institutions in modern society. Given the limits of therapy and its lag behind advances in scientific knowledge, much of AIDS work has been restricted to prevention and, consequently, to social practices. Paradoxically, many of today's doctors—at least those who now devote nearly all their energy to this new cause—seem to be playing a role from the past. Although they resemble hygienists who, during their heyday in nineteenth-century France, intervened in the name of health in all areas of life, they differ in a major way: most of them have avoided being used as a means of social control, as had often happened when hygienics was triumphant in dealing with tuberculosis and syphilis. Instead, most doctors have been the allies of patients and, even more, of the groups striving against discrimination and stigmatization, which were to be feared given instances of panic and efforts to exploit them politically.

Doctors and scientists have not worked alone. They have had to coordinate actions and negotiate with other partners. AIDS has exposed the limits of their autonomy, which has been conceptualized in sociology (Freidson 1970) as the medical profession's total freedom to define and control, by itself, the contents and terms of its practice of medicine. Starting in 1985, as French authorities began reacting and AIDS turned into a social issue, various groups and institutions became active. The press too played a stronger role. No longer just a stage from which various opinions were voiced, it became an actor in the debate as well as one of the issues to be debated: actions and discourses were organized as a function of the media. In October 1985, Nirascou in *Le Figaro* wrote, "AIDS is the first 'mediatic' illness." It is also the first illness to have created such tight and complicated relations between political authorities, doctors, scientists, and associations—relations mediated/mediatized by press and television.

VOLUNTEER ORGANIZATIONS IN THE CAMPAIGN AGAINST AIDS

Volunteer groups for helping PWAs soon took the forefront and placed patients on center stage. Inspired by the first associations created in the United States in 1982, especially by the Gay Men's Health Crisis (GMHC) (which the media had reported on), AIDES was formed in 1984 in France. In both countries, the most active persons at the origin of most of these initiatives were homosexuals. In fact, exchanges took place between organizations in the two countries. ARCAT-SIDA started bringing out an AIDS newsletter in 1989. Act-Up now exists in France. These are the most widely known AIDS organizations. From the start, before they were well formed and while they still had few members, they gathered and diffused information. They also tried to raise money for research, provide material and psychological support to the ill, and pressure the government as well as public opinion to intensify the AIDS campaign.

Several aspects of this activism are noteworthy. In a way, these organizations are an extension of the idea of patient groups, which had formed for various chronic illnesses (for example, diabetes, hemophilia, or renal failure). Even before AIDS, informal self-help groups had not limited themselves to creating bonds between persons suffering from the same illness. Refusing to be passive patients in the hands of the medical profession, their members sought to be actively involved in taking care of themselves on an equal footing with doctors. However, activist AIDS groups became full-fledged organizations. Their help has been an effective, crucial part of the care provided to PWAs. They have caused major changes in patients' relations with the medical profession and institutions. These relations range from a partnership between researchers, doctors, and patients for experimenting with certain drugs to violent criticism of medical professionals' shortcomings. These organizations refuse to be auxiliaries. They provide essential support to disadvantaged patients; but in France, Social Security pays all medical costs, and AZT can be obtained free of charge in hospitals. This situation is far different from in many countries, particularly the United States.

The issues raised by volunteer organizations' participation in health care reach beyond the illness itself. According to Defert (1989), president and founder of AIDES, AIDS more than any other illness has highlighted

the medical system's limits in backing its technical interventions up with support arrangements... In this vacuum, the self-organization of patients' cultural environment, a substitute for the family environment, has taken on full significance."

Furthermore, these organizations actively intervene in problems that may pit collective interests against individual rights (such as the consent for and confidentiality of testing) or lead to redefining expectations about the roles of the government, families, and citizens. They have gone so far as to define patients as social reformers. Having acquired considerable recognition and legitimacy, they have representatives sitting on national and international AIDS meetings, committees, conferences, and even the congresses convened by scientists, governments, or the WHO.

This activism does not keep us from glimpsing the shortcomings of and breaches in these organizations. After analyzing the importance of GMHC and ACT UP, Ouellette Kobasa (1990) pointed out the difficulties they have encountered: the tension between, on the one hand, their origins as fully democratic and participative voluntary associations working closely with PWAs and, on the other, their gradual institutionalization owing to growth and success. Little by little, hierarchies are forming, and the core group of leaders is being separated from other members, who become employees and are treated as such. Bureaucratic procedures are interfering with relations between volunteers and PWAs. Various studies (Pollak and Rosman 1989) carried out in France have shown that the situation here is not all that different. In fact, this general process occurs in the evolution of all voluntary associations (Sills 1968). Furthermore, these associations have ambivalent relations with the state. They were formed to make up for the lack of government action, and overall, they have been amazingly successful. Nonetheless, the state allocates funds to them. Conflicts thus break out, and accusations sometimes fly, as the organizations claim the government is trying to recuperate their activities or accuse each other of being too progovernmental (see Edelmann [1990] for debates during the International AIDS Conference organized by nongovernmental organizations in Paris).

CONCLUSION: AIDS AND THE SOCIAL SCIENCES

Just as AIDS has exposed the shortcomings of our medical system, the slowness of political decision making and breaches in our social organization, has it not also made the social sciences, in particular sociology, take a more critical look at themselves? These sciences have played a part in AIDS research: within a few years, several publications about AIDS have come out and every academic journal has devoted a special issue to this topic. The French case can be used to raise questions that can be asked of other cases. First, how have the social sciences been involved in AIDS research, and what can be expected of this involvement? Second, what impact will this new subject of study have on the social sciences—on their contents, approaches, and evolution?

In France, major efforts have been made in research since 1988 and the creation of the National Agency of AIDS Research. One of this agency's five research committees is devoted to the "human and social sciences." This is a noteworthy innovation in France where, unlike in English-speaking countries, medical sociology developed not in medical schools and medical research institutions but in university sociology departments and social-science research centers. In fact, all social-science disciplines—psychology, anthropology, economics, law, and history as well—have been involved in AIDS-related research. Many of these scholars, regardless of their discipline, had never worked before on problems having to do with illness or medicine. For this reason, the often excessive specialization, or compartmentalization, of medical sociologists may be overcome, and a real debate may take place among the disciplines interested in this new field of research. For example, a survey of the sexual behavior of 20,000 French persons is now being carried out not only by epidemiologist and public-health doctors but also by sociologists, social psychologists, demographers, psychoanalysts, and anthropologists.

The social sciences are indeed involved in many ways in AIDS-related research, but what are the limits and meaning of this involvement? Might it be mere lip service with no consequences? Do the results of such research have any chance of being taken into account when public policies are drawn up or when social reactions to the epidemic have to be handled? It is too early (and hard) to answer these questions. Of course, social scientists are active in the volunteer organizations, and their participation has affected the latter, which have borrowed knowledge, arguments, and conceptual frameworks from the social sciences.

But this involvement has taken place in a context where the medical and biological sciences have been relatively unable to solve problems related to the AIDS epidemic. Internationally, emphasis has been laid on modifying or preventing certain behaviors, and public authorities have turned toward the social sciences with this in mind. Despite their contributions to this research, the social sciences have shown that behaviors cannot be easily modified and that such modifications are not, by themselves, a means of stopping the epidemic from spreading. Can this boomerang on these sciences? Besides, what does it mean to have asked these disciplines to become involved in a context where other sciences, and authorities, have proven helpless? And might this involvement not also be useful in contexts where medicine is efficacious?

Although the social sciences can build up knowledge about how to manage both illness and patients' experiences in medical institutions, their involvement in AIDS research draws attention to their shortcomings. In France, most studies have concentrated on the general population, in particular young people. Research has focused on the psychosocial aspects of information campaigns, the image of AIDS, and perceptions of risk. Few studies have been conducted about PWAs and the health professionals who care for them. Social scientists have difficulty studying the painful experiences of illness and death, which present a problem for the whole society.

How has AIDS affected the contents of the social sciences? AIDS-related research should broaden the perspectives of the sociology of illness. AIDS has made sociologists turn to history in order to examine the notion of epidemic; they have learned to place patient care and health policy in a historical perspective. Moreover, AIDS and its management in daily life raise all the problems that crop up during chronic illnesses—problems having to do with the management of uncertainty, stigmatization, patients' careers, and the biographical aspects of illness as the patient's identity is reshaped (Siegel and Krauss 1991). Given AIDS' impact on society, and thanks to the "live" observation of the course of this new illness and the simultaneous involvement of all the social sciences in research, progress should be made in understanding the relations between micro- and macrosocial levels as well as in analyzing the feedback between individual experiences, cultural factors, and macrosocial structures. As Frankenberg (1986), an anthropologist, has noted, every patient's individual experience of illness (for instance of stigmatization) confronts him or her with the images produced and imposed by society. Behaviors are situated on a deep time-scale that reaches back to the bygone "afflictions" studied by historians. Reactions cannot be understood if we fail to look at the resources and limits of the health system in each country and of the health policies adopted by each government—at conceptions of solidarity and the way they are realized. These aspects are present in all illnesses, but we usually try to ignore them. They are more clearly present in the AIDS social phenomenon and may, therefore, be more easily perceived and understood.

ACKNOWLEDGMENT

This paper was translated from the French by Noal Mellott, Centre National de la Recherche Scientifique, Paris.

NOTES

1. In "Seeing the AIDS Patient" (Gilman 1988, ch. 14), the transition from bygone to modern representations of illness can be seen as reproductions of old engravings, and paintings of persons suffering from venereal disease, yield to photographs of PWAs.

2. Our study of how the AIDS social phenomenon has been constructed in France is based on an analysis of the 412 articles (or series) run in six French dailies from January 1982 to July 1986, in other words, during the time from the first publication of an article on AIDS till the Second International AIDS Conference, held in Paris on June 23-25, 1986. There were several reasons for choosing these six newspapers (*Le Figaro, L'Humanité, Libération, Le Matin, Le Monde, and Le Quotidien de Paris*). They have a national circulation and represent the positions of the major political forces present in France. Furthermore, each of them has a specialized journalist (sometimes a doctor) who regularly covers the medical field (Herzlich and Pierret 1988, 1989).

3. For example, compensation for HIV-positive hemophiliacs was discussed for years before a decision was reached in July 1989. In 1991 and 1992, the infection of hemophiliacs by HIV has created a major crisis in France. The delays in medical, administrative, and governmental reactions have been stressed. This point underlines the paradoxical character of AIDS: even if mobilization on this health problem has been exceptionally large, it appeared as insufficient.

REFERENCES

Berger, P. and T. Luckmann. 1966. *The Social Construction of Reality.* Garden City, NY: Doubleday.

Blaudin de Thé, G. 1984. "Les parias se mobilisent. A New York, la 'Gay Men Health Crisis' mène la lutte." *Le Monde* (26-27 Février).

Bourdelais, P. 1989. "Contagions d'hier et d'aujourd'hui." *Sciences Sociales et Santé : Sociétés à l'épreuve du sida* VII-(1, Special Issue): 12-17.

Bourdelais, P. and J.Y. Raulot. 1987. *Une peur bleue. Histoire du choléra en France.* Paris: Payot.

Brunet, J.B., G. David, P. Lantrade, A. Laporte, R. Salaman, D. Schwartz, and A.J. Valleron. 1990. "La prévalence de l'infection par le VIH en France en 1989." *Bulletin Epidémiologique Hebdomadaire* 37.

"Ce mal étrange qui frappe les homosexuels." 1982. *Le Quotidien de Paris* (6 Janvier).

Conan, E. 1982a. "Mystérieux cancer chez les homosexuels américains." *Libération* (6 Janvier).

_____. 1982b. "Le mal mystérieux des homosexuels américains (suite)." *Libération* (6-7 Février).

Defert, D. 1989. "Le malade réformateur social." *Gai-Pied Hebdo* 29(June): 58-61.

Delumeau, J. and Y. Lequin, eds. 1987. *Les malheurs du temps.* Paris: Larousse.

Edelmann, F. 1990. "Les raisons d'un boycottage." *Le Monde* (November 4/5).

Escoffier-Lambiotte, C. 1982. "Drogue, Virus et défense immunitaire. Une mystérieuse épidémie au Etats-Unis." *Le Monde* (27 Janvier).

Fox, R. 1959. *Experiment Perilous: Physicians and Patients Facing the Unknown.* Glencoe, IL: Free Press of Glencoe.

Frankenberg, R. 1986. "Sickness as Cultural Performance: Drama, Trajectory and Pilgrimage, Root Metaphors and the Making Social of Disease." *International Journal of Health Services* XVI(4): 603-626.

Freidson, E. 1970. *Profession of Medicine.* New York: Dodd, Mead.

Gilman, S. 1988. *Disease and Representation: Images of Illness from Madness to AIDS.* Ithaca, NY: Cornell University Press.

Goody, J. 1977. *The Domestication of the Savage Mind.* Cambridge: Cambridge University Press.

Grmek, M. 1989. *Histoire du sida.* Paris: Payot.

Herzlich, C. and J. Pierret, 1987. *Illness and Self in Society.* Baltimore, MD: The John Hopkins University Press. (English translation of *Malades d'hier, malades d'aujourd'hui.* Paris: Payot, 1984.)

————. 1988 "Une maladie dans L'espace public. Le SIDA dans six quotidiens français." *Annales ESC* 5: 1109-1134.

————. 1989 "The Construction of a Social Phenomenon: AIDS in the French Press." *Social Science and Medicine* XXIX(11): 1235-1242.

Latour, B. 1985. "Les 'vues' de l'esprit." *Culture technique* 14: 4-29.

Mann, J., J. Chin, P. Piot, and T. Quinn. 1988. "Le sida dans le monde." *Pour la science* 143: 56-65.

Nirascou, G. 1985. "Optimisme mesuré." *Le Figaro* (30 Octobre).

Ouellette Kobasa, S. 1990. "AIDS and Volunteer Associations: Perspectives on Social and Individual Change." *The Milbank Quarterly* LXVIII(2): 280-294.

Pollak, M. 1988. *Les homosexuels et le sida. Sociologie d'une épidémie.* Paris: A.M. Métailié.

Pollak, M., W. Dab, and J.P. Moatti. 1989. "Systèmes de réaction au sida et action préventive." *Sciences Sociales et Santé: "Sociétés à l'épreuve du sida "* VII (1, Special Issue): 111-140.

Pollak, M. and S. Rosman, 1989. "Les associations de lutte contre le sida: éléments d'évaluation et de réflexion," MIRE-EHESS-CNRS research report, July.

Pauwels, L. 1986. Editorial. *Figaro-Magazine* (6 Décembre).

Rozenberg, C. 1989. "What Is an Epidemic? AIDS in Historical Perspective." *Daedalus* CXVIII(2): 1-17.

Sauclières, G. 1982. "La pneumonie des homosexuels." *La Recherche* 131: 392-393.

Siegel, K. and B. Krauss, 1991. "Living with HIV Infection: Adaptive Tasks of Seropositive Gay Men." *Journal of Health and Social Behavior* XXXII(3): 17-32.

Sills, D. 1968. "Voluntary Associations." Pp. 357-378 in *International Encyclopedia of the Social Sciences.* New York: MacMillan.

Szafran, M. 1983. "Quand une maladie devient malédiction. Aux Etats-Unis, les nouveaux puritains proclament que le sida est une juste punition." *Le Matin* (21 Juin).

Veron, E. 1981. *Construire l'événement.* Paris: Editions de Minuit.

Vigy, M. 1983. "Alerte au syndrome 'gay.' " *Le Figaro* (22 Mars).

Weitz, R. 1989. "Uncertainty and the Lives of Persons with AIDS." *Journal of Health and Social Behavior* 3: 270-281.

THE PUBLIC AND PERSONAL
MEANINGS OF BISEXUALITY IN
THE CONTEXT OF AIDS

Mary Boulton and Ray Fitzpatrick

ABSTRACT

Throughout the AIDS epidemic in the United Kingdom and United States, men who have sex with men have constituted the largest group with HIV infection and AIDS. Studies carried out among this population, however, have found that a small but significant proportion are also sexually active with women. The recognition that HIV could be transmitted through both homosexual and heterosexual sex has drawn attention to this hitherto shadowy social category of bisexual men as a potential bridging group between gay men and the rest of the population. From a public-health perspective, it has become important to enumerate and describe the behavior of bisexual men and to develop appropriate health-education programes. However, in both epidemiological and behavioral research, problems in defining and describing the phenomenon have arisen from poorly conceptualizing and distinguishing among different aspects of sexuality. Similarly, health-education programs have been limited by a lack of understanding of the nature and meaning of bisexuality. This paper draws on

The Social and Behavioral Aspects of AIDS.
Advances in Medical Sociology, Volume 3, pages 77-100.
Copyright © 1993 by JAI Press Inc.
ISBN: 1-55938-439-5

two studies, one of homosexually active men and one of bisexual men, to explore the relationship between self-ascribed sexual orientation and sexual behavior and the meanings they have to the men themselves. This analysis points to the problematic nature of approaches to sexuality based on the essentialist concept of sexual identity. The majority of men who have sex with both men and women do not describe or account for themselves and their lives in terms of a bisexual identity. The category of bisexual has come to prominence because of the central role of sexual behavior in the transmission of HIV. Bisexuality in turn underlines the importance of reconceptualizing sexuality in terms of relationships between individuals rather than the essence within the individual, and of shifting research attention to the social and interactionist nature of sexual encounters. Such a shift also calls into question the notion of bisexual men as a distinct and identifiable group within the sexually active population.

INTRODUCTION

By the time that AIDS was first recognized as a syndrome, some twenty years of successful political pressures to increase personal rights had resulted in a quite well-defined public identity for gay men. Thus when, in the language of epidemiology, homosexual males were identified as a major risk group for HIV infection in both the United States and the United Kingdom, public discourse had a number of clearly formed images and stereotypes by means of which to interpret the emerging epidemic. Initial medical terminology referring to "Gay Related Immune Disease" (GRID) was paralleled by popular media discussion of the "gay plague." The most organized initial response in terms of education and prevention came from sections of the "gay community." When the sexual mechanisms of transmission of the virus, particularly penetrative anal intercourse, were clearly demonstrated, the importance of sexuality to the AIDS epidemic was fully established. However, at every level from medical research to popular imagination, this early phase raised issues of "gay" sexuality.

Slowly at first, but accelerated in the United Kingdom by national health-education programs, awareness grew that heterosexual sex might also transmit the virus. At this point a somewhat shadowy social category—bisexuals—came into focus. Studies carried out among the gay population found that a small but significant proportion of men were also sexually active with women (Fitzpatrick, Hart, Boulton, McLean, and Dawson 1989). Men who had sex with both men and women were seen as constituting a bridging group between gay men and the rest of the population. From the perspective of public health and its functions of predicting and controlling the AIDS epidemic, it became important to enumerate and describe the behavior of bisexual men and to develop appropriate health-education programs. However, in both the United States and the United Kingdom, official statistics of the epidemic as well as virtually all epidemiological and behavioral research have tended to view homosexual and bisexual men as one category for such purposes as presenting prevalence rates of AIDS and HIV and describing the behavior of at-risk groups. This categorization reflects a more widespread inability to see important distinctions between homosexual and bisexual. The two terms were viewed as one in medical classifications based on the mechanisms of transmission of the virus. The readiness with which homosexual and bisexual men were subsumed in AIDS data may also have reflected broader assumptions of the unity of a socially deviant group. There had been no widespread or organized equivalent of the gay liberation movements of the 1960s and 1970s to establish bisexuality in the public consciousness. Academic research was not well placed to fill the vacuum in the public's understanding since far less systematic attention had been given to bisexual men compared with the now substantial social-scientific literature on gay men and the gay community.

This paper examines how bisexual men have been treated in epidemiological and behavioral research in relation to AIDS to date. It will become clear how poorly described and distinguished are the range of behaviors that include homosexual and bisexual sexuality. Many problems arise from poorly distinguishing sexual behavior from self-ascribed sexual orientation, sexual preferences or other aspects of sexuality. Evidence is reviewed that male bisexual sexual behavior may arise in a remarkably diverse range of social contexts and may encompass a diverse range of sexual histories. We then draw on two studies of homosexual and bisexual behavior conducted by us and other colleagues to show that the relationship between self-ascribed sexual orientation and sexual behavior in this field is complex. The first study is a large-scale, longitudinal survey of homosexually active men which demonstrates that the individual's view of his sexual orientation does not neatly map onto his sexual behavior either at one point in time or predictively over time. This raises the general question of what bisexuality means to individuals. The second study is a smaller, qualitative study of men with recent bisexual sexual histories in which this issue is explored. A major theme in the men's accounts concerns the dilemmas and decisions they confront regarding disclosure of their sexuality to significant others. Faced with a public view of bisexuality as anomalous, deviant, or indeed nonexistent, men in this situation continuously have to cope with an already socially stigmatized identity. Uncertainties about sexual boundaries and definitions in the public domain are thus paralleled by and interconnected with private and personal uncertainties.

Overall, the paper therefore addresses a category that has proved shadowy and elusive at two quite different levels. At the level of scientific knowledge of the AIDS epidemic, the distinctive role of bisexual men constitutes a major challenge to researchers at very basic levels of defining, let alone discovering and describing the phenomenon. These problems ultimately reflect the complexities of decisions about how to define sexuality to self and to significant others faced by individuals with bisexual sexual histories.

BISEXUALITY AS AN EPIDEMIOLOGICAL PROBLEM

The public-health perspective requires that the size of the bisexual male population be estimated and types of sexual behavior be described in order to provide models and predictions of the development of the AIDS epidemic. As with all questions of the sexual behavior of human populations, very little contemporary and systematic data exist to provide an answer and what does exist gives a very variable picture. In the United Kingdom, despite official governmental disapproval, a national survey of the sexual lifestyles of a random sample of the British population was conducted in 1990-1991 and will soon report its results. However a pilot study for the main survey (Johnson et al. 1989) reported that only two men (0.6% of male respondents) maintained that they had ever had sex with another man. Both also reported female partners. The investigators express doubts as to whether this low figure reflects reluctance to admit homosexual sexual behavior in the context of a survey. One of the few other national random surveys, conducted in Norway, produced a very different estimate (Sundet, Kvalem, Magnus, and Bakketeig 1988) with 3 percent of men reporting *ever* having had both male and female sexual partners. With a slightly different criterion for bisexuality, an Australian survey found 4.2 percent of currently married men had had a male sexual partner *in the previous year* (Ross 1988).

Surveys of sexual behavior in random samples of the population are politically contentious and difficult to conduct. In many ways, gay men have been far more prepared to discuss issues of sexual behavior in the waves of behavioral research that have followed the AIDS epidemic. Nonclinic community surveys of homosexually active men produce a range of estimates for bisexual behavior. Thus, one survey of gay men in England (McManus and McEvoy 1987) reported that just under 5 percent of gay men also reported a current female partner. By contrast, a second survey of homosexually active men found that 10 percent reported a female sexual partner in the previous year, and 58 percent had had a female sexual partner at least once in their lifetime (Fitzpatrick, Hart, Boulton, McLean, and Dawson 1989). A government-sponsored survey of gay men conducted in gay clubs and pubs to monitor the impact of health education found that the frequency with which men reported at least one female sexual partner in the previous year varied across three different waves of interviews between 27 percent and 32 percent (Department of Health and Social Security 1987). Similar variation has been found in North American and Australian surveys of gay men.

One of the commonest sources of data about bisexual men are surveys of attenders at sexually transmitted diseases clinics. On common-sense grounds, clinic attenders are likely to be more sexually active than the general population, so general inferences are difficult. Moreover, clinic reports tend not to be clear about criteria for assigning individuals to sexual categories or frequently collapse the distinction between homosexual and bisexual men. Nevertheless some estimates are available. A few studies report the proportions of all attenders who are bisexual men. Two different Danish clinics produced remarkably different estimates 7 percent and 28 percent (Boulton and Weatherburn 1990). By contrast, the Collaborative Study Group of consultants in genitourinary medicine (1989) produced estimates for two consecutive years of the proportion of homosexually active men attending the clinics of 16 different towns in England who were bisexual—19 percent and 24 percent. A more detailed investigation in one very large London clinic (Evans et al. 1989) reported that the proportions of gay men who reported a female partner were 9 percent in relation to the last six months, 11 percent in relation to the last year, and 29 percent in relation to the last five-year period.

It is hardly surprising, in view of the above variability of evidence, that when, in response to the AIDS epidemic, efforts have been made to describe the kinds of sexual practices associated with bisexual men (particularly those that might be relevant to HIV transmission), the picture has also proved quite unclear. Thus, it is not clear how similar or different are rates of penetrative anal sex in bisexual compared with homosexual men, how readily "safer sex" has been adopted; and whether there are distinctive patterns of heterosexual sexual behavior found in bisexual men (Fitzpatrick, Hart, Boulton, McLean, and Dawson 1989).

A number of simple but fundamental points are bound to strike the reader from even a cursory review of epidemiological and behavioral surveys. First, there are wide variations in estimates of the proportion of men who are bisexual. Second, the operational definitions of bisexual male sexual behavior also vary between studies. At the extreme, definitions vary from use of self-ascribed orientation ("bisexual") to behavioral definitions (e.g., sex with a male and female in a given time period). Third, there is a great deal of variation between behavioral definitions in terms of the time period covered in which sex with both a male and female sexual partner is counted as indicating bisexual behavior. Indeed, operational definitions vary as much as the estimates they generate. Furthermore, there is nothing particularly meaningful about any one definition compared with another. An operational definition of bisexual men as "men who say they are *gay* and have had sex with another woman in the last five years" is not an inherently more or less convincing or meaningful definition than, say, "men who have had sex with a man and a woman in the last two years." It might be argued that there is nothing particularly remarkable about the apparent arbitrariness and variability of operational definitions of bisexuality. Like many other subjects of study in epidemiology, the parameter of sex with men and women is one that emerges from epidemiological concerns such as the mathematical modeling of HIV infection from patterns of sexual behavior rather than reflecting social constructs *out there* that might be expected to reflect meaningful social categories. Indeed, the particular uses of behavioral data in epidemiology necessitate an essentially arbitrary operational language.

Our view of this operational approach to bisexuality would be that it reveals something more basic than the requirements of epidemiological research. There exists a very powerful dichotomous language of homosexual versus heterosexual, gay versus straight. This language both reflects and reinforces an essentialist view of these polar sexual categories. Moreover, all too frequently essentialist language has collapsed distinctions so that gay and homosexual become equated in the epidemiology of AIDS. By contrast, bisexual lacks a clear place in the dichotomous language of sexual preference. There are men, as our data will illustrate, who view bisexuality as a distinct essence. For the public discourse of AIDS however, the term wavers between, on the one hand, merger with homosexuality on the basis of a unified risk of transmission category and shared minority deviance and, on the other hand, a no-mans-land of operational arbitrariness.

Prior to AIDS, a nascent sociology of sexuality, while focusing on gay and homosexual lifestyles, had begun to acknowledge the phenomenon of bisexuality. The bisexual was viewed as "somehow outside the conventional sexual categories" (Paul 1983/1984, p. 53) and socially marginal; a "conceptual loose-end" in a "precarious niche" (Blumstein and Schwartz 1977, p. 31), and a scientific problem that "resists being easily categorized" (Gagnon 1989, p. 59). More commonly, bisexuality was subsumed under the more significant category of homosexuality or viewed as psychopathological abnormality.

VARIETIES OF MALE BISEXUALITY

It is now clear that it would be more accurate to refer to male *bisexualities*. Gagnon (1989) distinguishes between six different contexts in which men may have sex with both a male and female partner. One category is men who lead heterosexual lives but also earn money as homosexual prostitutes. A second group are men who again lead heterosexual lives but, because of the limitations imposed by prison life, have homosexual sex. This situational category could be extended to other same-sex institutions such as boarding schools or the armed services, although legal constraints make such situational bisexuality very difficult to document (Boulton and Weatherburn 1990).

A very different, third context of male bisexual behavior is that of men who are married but have secretive and anonymous homosexual sex, most often in public places such as parks or toilets. Quite different again is the fourth category found in Latin American cultures, in which the man who is the active inserter in homosexual sex continues to think of himself as a man and heterosexual whereas the passive partner in anal intercourse is culturally defined as a woman. Less well-described is a fifth context of bisexuality identified in heterosexual men "messing around" homosexually under the effects of alcohol or drug use, where sexual access to females is not available.

Men in most of the above contexts continue to view themselves in conventional heterosexual terms. Only from an observer's perspective may their behavior lead them to be labelled bisexual. However, there is now a small, sixth social category of men who have a clear and distinctive view of themselves as being sexually attracted to both men and women. These men are far more likely to select "bisexual" to describe themselves and to acknowledge a distinctive sexual lifestyle. Although poorly documented, some men have become involved in "out" social groups with other bisexual men and women to support and promote bisexual lifestyles.

Gagnon's typology of male bisexualities is based on social contexts and draws attention to the very varied circumstances in which bisexuality may occur. We want to add an additional typology of bisexualities that emerges if one recognizes the essential dimension of *time*. For most of the bisexual men whom our study has investigated, bisexuality emerges from their *sexual histories*. Different sequences of sexual biography can be described in terms of different types of bisexuality. For some men that we interviewed, bisexual sexual behavior was seen as a *transitional phase* between a heterosexual past and a gay present and future. A second pattern we term *serial*. This appears to be a less common sexual history associated with younger men who had relatively few partners of either sex. These men alternate between nonoverlapping phases of homosexual and heterosexual activity. A third pattern involves a *unique deviation* from usual sexual relations. A number of men described themselves as having established heterosexual or homosexual lives but then having one or two sexual involvements of the opposite kind. For some, this deviant episode arose under the special circumstances of disinhibiting effects of alcohol or drugs, for others from giving physical expression to one special friendship. Finally and most commonly there is a pattern of *concurrent bisexuality* in which men are involved in substantial overlapping homosexual and heterosexual sexual activities. Thus, whether referring to varying social contexts or to the different sexual histories of bisexuality, it is clear that a very diverse range of experiences is included by the term.

SEXUAL BEHAVIOR, SEXUAL ATTRACTION, AND SEXUAL IDENTITY

This diversity of experience behind the category bisexual can also be noted at an individual level. There are a number of different components and levels to individuals' sexuality. Although acknowledged in the psychoanalytic and (some) psychological literature and given emphasis in the work of Kinsey, the dimensionality of sexuality has yet to be more widely recognised. The experiences of male bisexuals clearly point in this direction. Some of the complexities of sexuality in relation to bisexual behavior can be seen in a longitudinal study we carried out to investigate homosexually active men's responses to the AIDS epidemic in England (Fitzpatrick, Hart, Boulton, McLean, and Dawson 1989; Fitzpatrick, McLean, Boulton, Hart, and Dawson 1990). This study involved a sample of 502 men recruited in a number of different cities in England through gay clubs, pubs, and organizations, from sexually transmitted disease clinics, and by snowball sampling. The criterion for inclusion in the study was that the man had had sex with another man in the previous five years. The study was in the form of structured interviews, a substantial section of which focused on detailed sexual histories. The sample comprised fairly young men; mean age was 31.6 years (*SD* 10.4) with a range from 16 to 67. Like most studies of gay and homosexual males, the men were well-educated; 63 percent had received some form of higher education (university, polytechnic, or further education college).

Of the sample of 502 homosexually active men, 58 (11.6%) had also had some kind of sex with a female partner in the year prior to the interview. Men were also asked to place themselves in terms of their sexual fantasies and attractions on the Kinsey scale which has a range of seven points, from "exclusively heterosexual" (point 0) through "equally heterosexual and homosexual" (point 3), to "exclusively homosexual" (point 6). Two issues of interest emerge from comparing the results of the behavioral information with men's description of sexual attractions. First, 30 percent (133/444) of those who had not had sex with a female partner nevertheless described some degree of attraction to women. Conversely, 12 percent (7/58) of those who had had a female sexual partner in the previous year described themselves as exclusively homosexual in terms of sexual attractions.

Similarly, sexual behavior may be related to self-ascribed sexual orientation. Men were asked to select the word or phrase that best described their sexual orientation. Seventy-eight percent described themselves as gay, 9 percent preferred the term homosexual, 10 percent selected bisexual, and the remaining 2 percent selected unique terms such as transvestite. Of the 58 men who had had sex with both men and women in the previous year, 33 (57%) selected "bisexual" to describe themselves. However, the remaining 25 men (43%) preferred the designation "gay" or some other unique term. In the same way, there are discrepancies between self-ascribed sexual orientation and how individuals described their sexual fantasies and attractions. In particular, of the 392 men who referred to themselves as gay, 105 (27%) chose a point on the Kinsey scale that indicated their homosexuality was combined with some degree of heterosexual attraction.

Another way of looking at this data would be to consider the epidemiological task of enumerating bisexual males. Altogether, 192 (38%) of this sample of homosexually active men refer to themselves as in some way bisexual, either in terms of sexual attractions, sexual orientation, or recent sexual behavior. However, only 33 men would be "captured" by all three criteria. The remaining 159 men either would or would not be included as bisexual men depending on the particular definition used. Furthermore, one criterion, sexual attractions on the Kinsey scale, would capture most of the men who were in some sense bisexual. Only 8/192 described their orientation or recent sexual behavior as bisexual but described their sexual attractions as solely homosexual. However, if a survey were to rely on the Kinsey scale to count bisexuality, the majority of men it would define as bisexual (i.e., 116/184) would neither have described themselves as bisexual in answer to a simple question about orientation, nor would have reported bisexual sexual behavior in the sense of sex with both a male or female partner in the previous year.

We followed up the sample by means of a postal questionnaire nine months after the initial interview. Three-hundred-and-sixty-nine (74%) of the original sample returned the questionnaire, a satisfactory response rate in view of the geographical mobility of the sample and the extensive steps we had had to adopt in guaranteeing the confidentiality and anonymity of respondents when they were first recruited into the study. The follow-up survey provided an opportunity to examine the stability of some aspects of bisexuality.

Eighty-eight individuals rated their behavior as to some degree bisexual on the Kinsey scale, either at the initial interview or at follow-up. However, the relative instability of this rating is indicated by the fact that only 34/88 (39%) were consistent across the two assessments. The majority (61%) rated their behavior as to some degree heterosexual and homosexual on one occasion while switching to a rating of exclusively homosexual on the other occasion. Similarly, men were asked to answer some detailed questions about sexual behavior in the follow-up questionnaire. Overall, 46 men reported having sex with a male and a female partner in the previous year, in at least one of the two assessments. Again, only 14/46 (30%) consistently reported this bisexual sexual behavior on both occasions. Finally, men were asked in the questionnaire to choose the word or phrase that best described their sexual orientation. Thirty-nine of the sample described themselves as bisexual on at least one of the two occasions, but only 20 (51%) elected to describe themselves this way on both occasions.

BISEXUAL MEN: A FOCUSED STUDY

Thus, survey research can be quite revealing. It indicates that male bisexuality is multidimensional, involving at least three distinct components of fantasies and attractions, sexual orientation, and sexual behavior. A second study was initiated to investigate in more depth bisexual mens' sexual behavior and self-conception in relation to AIDS (Boulton, Schramm-Evans, Fitzpatrick, and Hart 1991). A sample of 60 bisexual men was recruited via bisexual groups based in Edinburgh and London, via advertisements placed in appropriate magazines, and finally via sexually transmitted diseases clinics. The criterion for recruitment into the study was sexual contact with both men and women at some time in the previous five years. The study was in the form of a semi-structured interview which included both open-ended and fixed-choice questions. The sample comprised fairly young, middle-class men; mean age was 34 years with a range from 19 to 71 and 65 percent had non-manual occupations.

Although all of the men were behaviorally bisexual by our criterion, only one-half described themselves by use of this term. About a quarter described themselves as gay and the rest used a variety of terms including straight, normal, and unrestrained. Similarly, only just over half had had both male and female partners in the year prior to interview. A quarter had had male partners only and a fifth had had female partners only. Using the Kinsey scale, however, 95 percent described their fantasies and attractions as to some degree both homosexual and heterosexual.

PERCEPTIONS OF BISEXUALITY

Men were first asked how they thought the public viewed bisexuality. Virtually all the men in the sample thought that there was little awareness of, and hence little concern about, bisexuality among the general public. As one man said:

> Most of the public are clueless. They have no idea about bisexuality. They have a very clear perception now of gay men as a group. Gay men have made themselves socially very visible. Bisexual men are less visible. If they are seen at all it's as "non-straight."

Little distinction was made between homosexuals and bisexuals, any same-sex activity putting the individual firmly into the category of homosexual. Homosexuality was frowned on and, insofar as bisexuality entailed homosexuality, it too was stigmatized. But prior to AIDS, bisexuality itself was not a concept with which the public was familiar nor was there any recognition of bisexuals as a discrete category within society. One of the consequences of HIV/AIDS, and the media interest and health-education campaigns surrounding it, has been to draw attention to bisexuality and to begin to differentiate bisexuals as a distinct category.

At the heart of this process of differentiation is the epidemiological description of bisexuals as a bridging group between the homosexual and heterosexual communities. Bisexuality is associated with HIV/AIDS and with the spread of the epidemic from "them" to "us." As several men pointed out, the image of HIV/AIDS as an unseen contagion, a threat from within, has provided the basis for an image of bisexuality itself which the public has readily taken up.

> Bisexual men are probably distrusted more than gay men, given the current climate. The idea that we are a bridging group between the gay and straight communities. We are expected to be kept at arms length. Also it goes deeper than AIDS. Supposedly straight men do feel more threatened by bisexual men than gay men. It isn't only AIDS that they spread to the straight community.

Bisexuals are seen as ill, weak, and unhappy in themselves but more significantly as deceptive and untrustworthy, morally corrupting and socially disruptive to others.

Men were then asked how they *personally* viewed bisexuality. Almost all the men indicated that, in their view, bisexuality was natural, normal, and common. Fifty one men (91%) thought that the potential for bisexuality was common or very common in the general population and 58 men (97%), that more people than realized it would enjoy sex with both men and women. They emphasized that most people had the potential for attraction to both men and women although these feelings were usually suppressed by social norms and social conditioning. Few people might behave bisexually, but the essence of bisexuality—of attraction to men and to women—was in most people:

> I think basically everybody is bisexual, just some people hide these or suppress these feelings and other people let them go. I think basically everybody is bisexual, there's a wee bit of bisexuality in everybody.

They saw their own sexual behavior in this light, as normal and right for them. Few could explain how they had come to be bisexual and indeed the notion of an explanation seemed inappropriate. None described any dramatic event which had precipitated their bisexuality nor did they feel that there was anything unusual about their circumstances which allowed them to pursue it. They stressed the similarity between themselves and other people. They differed only in having the *opportunity* to act on their attractions and the *confidence* to do so when the opportunity arose.

The majority of men had come to terms with their bisexuality and felt it was an expression of their true selves. Forty-seven men (78%) said that in an *ideal* world they would prefer to be bisexual and 46 men (78%) that they expected to continue to have sex with men and women. A number of men recognized the difficulties involved in bisexuality and only 37 (62%) said that in *this* world they would prefer to be bisexual. The problems of bisexuality were seen to arise largely from the attitudes of others, in a world where people were expected to be either heterosexual or homosexual but not both. Bisexual behavior was recognized as deviant even if it was not abnormal and the stresses of living a deviant lifestyle were acknowledged.

Although most of the men expected to continue to have male and female partners, bisexuality as such did not seem to provide an organizing principle in their lives. Only half the men (57%) described themselves as bisexual, and even those who did used the term more in a descriptive sense than an ideological sense:

> I would normally try to avoid labelling myself as much as labelling others, I suppose I thought, 'OK, obviously I've got homosexual tendencies to which I'm giving expression, and I've also got heterosexual tendencies and I'm having relations both ways, so perhaps I'm bisexual if I have to put a term on it.' I didn't go off and check what that meant in the dictionary. Expressing my sexuality was just one of many things I was wanting and doing at that time and since.

Bisexual groups have been established in London and Edinburgh and many gay societies have a bisexual interest group. These groups provide a reference point for behaviorally bisexual men and a focus for the development of a bisexual identity. Nine men were recruited from these bisexual groups. Of the remaining 51 men in the sample, however, only nine (18%) had had even passing contact with a bisexual group. The remaining 42 had had *no* contact at all, nor did they wish to have any. Moreover, only 12 of these 51 men (24%) felt that bisexuality could ever be a political issue for them, and even these men expressed little emotional commitment to the idea.

On a personal level, 38 men (63%) knew few or no bisexual men as friends and only three expressed any interest in meeting other bisexuals simply because they were bisexual:

> I like male company and I like female company. Whether or not they are bisexual makes no difference at all.

Only a few men actively sought out other bisexuals to support a bisexual identity and lifestyle. Indeed, most men took a fairly individualistic view of their sexuality and were primarily concerned with ensuring that they could continue to have both male and female partners. Since bisexuality is still largely unacceptable to others, they wanted to maintain a public identity as straight or, less often, as gay and would not have welcomed associations which marked them out as bisexual. Instead, they moved between the gay and straight communities, drawing on each as it suited them, and seemed to prefer doing so to joining a third, bisexual community. They felt little collective solidarity with other bisexuals and little concern with public acceptance of bisexuality so long as they could continue to have both male and female partners themselves.

MANAGING RELATIONSHIPS

In a society in which homosexual behavior is stigmatized in the general population and bisexuality rejected in the gay community, men who have sex with men and women may anticipate a hostile reaction from both male and female partners. They must therefore find a way of managing information about their past or present behavior in such a way that it does not threaten new or continuing relationships. The strategies developed to do so involve varying degrees of disclosure according, on the one hand, to the men's perceptions of what is likely to be acceptable to the partner and, on the other, to their commitment to sustaining the relationship. Different issues arise in relation to male and female partners, and men may adopt different strategies with partners of each sex. Similarly, casual and regular relationships raise different sorts of issues, which may be managed in different ways. The strategies which men may *prefer* to use depend largely on the extent of their own desire for openness about their sexuality and for acceptance of their sexuality by their partners. The "success" of their strategies depends more on external circumstances and the attitudes and experience of the partners concerned.

Male Partners

A sexual history which includes female partners was perceived as essentially acceptable to male partners. Heterosexuality is the norm in our society and social pressures are seen as pushing men into sexual relationships with women. Over half of homosexually active men have had sex with a woman at some time, so many of the men's male partners will also have had female partners. Thus most men expected that their male partners would find their behavior neither surprising nor repugnant nor particularly significant, and the management of information about this was not a major issue. Casual partners were assumed to be disinterested in any aspect of the men's sexual history but were told about female partners on the rare occasions that they asked:

If they ask I tell them. Most don't ask.

Henry knew because we met through a bisexual group. The others didn't because we didn't know each other long enough.

Regular partners were expected to be interested in previous partners as an aspect of their personal history and were usually told about female partners in this context:

> Some know, some don't. My friends know my sexual history with women. Others don't care.

Female Partmers

The men in the sample were aware that their sexual activities with men might not be acceptable to women who were also their sexual partners. Some thought that women would see them as not properly male or not sufficiently masculine to be proper partners:

> I expect women would be quite upset. I think, looked at in their terms, you might be perceived as not wholly male, because you have sex with other men as well, so from that point of view I would expect women to be upset. Especially in British culture, it's part of the stereotype of gay men.

Others indicated that women found the idea of sexual contact between men dirty or repulsive:

> They think it's disgusting, men together and especially anal sex. They think it's dirty.

> I should think it would make them sick. They would recoil in horror. It would be a terrible shock to them.

The AIDS epidemic was seen as feeding in to this, reinforcing the image of dirt and pollution and heightening the sense of fear and repulsion. A few men also thought that women looked on bisexual men as screwed up, untrustworthy or a bad risk because they were inherently incapable of settling into a monogamous relationship which most women were seen to want:

> I assume women see bisexuals as potential deceivers, people who would let them down in a relationship. People who can't make up their minds.

or as another man expressed it:

> The general view is that bisexuals get married but then go out and continue to have sex with men, so they make unsatisfactory husbands and fathers. Basically, they are not to be trusted.

For a variety reasons, then, a history of male partners was expected to be unacceptable to most female partners and the management of this information was taken very seriously. Moreover, current male partners were seen as unacceptable for additional reasons and information about such partners was seen as requiring particularly careful management. Strategies for managing information with female partners, were therefore, much more elaborated and differentiated than they were with male partners. Three quite different strategies, involving varying degrees of disclosure, could be identified in the men's accounts of their relationships.

Total Concealment

The First strategy was one of total concealment of any sexual contact with men:

> None of these women know I have ever had sex with men.

> No, my wife doesn't know, not to the best of my knowledge.

For some men, concealment was a deliberate strategy which they used for utilitarian reasons, that is, to maintain their sexual relationships with women:

> I would have thought that if my wife found out I was having sexual contact with men she would leave me immediately. If Jane or Sue knew they might blackmail me.

Some men stressed the importance of protecting others from information which would be hurtful to them:

> It would obviously upset her and it might diminish her own feelings of worth to me, that is the principle consideration.... I think either non-monogamy or male partners would be bad, unfaithfulness would be the main element, and the male part would just make it worse.

Such men went to great lengths to keep their relationships with men entirely separate from their relationships with women:

> I am expected home most evenings and all nights. So I am limited. If a man asked me to come round at a time I was expected at home I simply wouldn't go. I manage that by having a private mailing address. I would take someone's number but never ever give mine, nor do I carry letters around on my person or keep them at work or at home. Having to be discreet is the most frustrating thing. You become a sort of amateur Jekyll and Hyde. All my male partners know I'm married. They accept that limitation, otherwise it's not on.

For others, this deception was less complicated:

> It's made easier by the fact that one half of one's life is lived in London and the other half not, so that geographical divide makes it easier. I can well imagine that if I was self-employed and living above a shop, it would make it considerably more difficult. I mean you don't make these choices in your life, you have to judge them as they emerge. I can't honestly say it's been terribly difficult.

Other men were aware that their female partners did not know about their sexual activities with men but felt that they were not deliberately concealing the information. Their own sexual history was simply not an issue in their relationships with women. While they made no particular effort to disclose information about their male partners, they made no effort to conceal it either:

> We met on a training course and got on very well together. But we never got into the situation, sitting around in bars or hotels, of having deep discussions about people being gay or whatever. I didn't keep anything from her by lying, but she would have assumed that I was straight. I didn't actively keep anything from her, I never expected to sleep with her but we were both in her hotel room late at night, merry and it just happened. I didn't actively tell her any lies or mislead her.

As with male partners, casual relationships with female partners often presented little need nor opportunity for disclosure:

> With Kathy I don't think it would have gone down terribly well if I had said "Look I'm a gay man, shall we go to bed." If I had told her she wouldn't have gone to bed with me. But also, you don't sit down and have a deep conversation with someone when you're drunk at a party. It just happens, you're in bed together.

Partial Disclosure

The second strategy in the management of information about male sexual partners was one of partial disclosure, that is, disclosure of information about male sexual partners in the past. For some, this was a passive strategy, in that it involved only acknowledging what the women already knew:

> She knew beforehand, I didn't have to tell her anything. She is bisexual too.

For others, it was a more deliberate strategy, in which the men ensured that their female partners were aware that they had had male partners in the past. This often involved explicit discussions of past sexual history:

> June knew before the relationship started. She already knew from someone else, and I told her to make sure she knew before the relationship actually started, I thought I'd try the honesty bit from the start rather than wait until the end and it worked because she accepted me for what I was without anything else. She took it as though it was a normal part of life. She already had several gay friends. I told her that I had slept with men and that I had had sex with men and that I had lots of feelings towards men. I told her about the past.

As the latter quote suggests, some men felt it important to tell their female partners about their previous male partners as part of establishing an open, honest, trusting relationship between them. These men seemed to want to be accepted for who they were and to have their sense of themselves confirmed and validated by their female partners. Other men appeared to have more cynical reasons for telling their female partners about their bisexuality, letting them know from the beginning where they stood and preparing the ground for male partners in the future:

> Annie asked out of curiosity more than anything. She knew I was living with my male partner, one of these unstated things, I didn't actually say so. My second wife has "esp." I said I was gay, I didn't tell her I was having lots of other casual partners. I couldn't deny it. My homosexual inclinations meant that sooner or later she would have found out. It was better to let her know from the outset just exactly what she was letting herself in for.

When their relationships with women were relatively brief, there was no time for the men to have concurrent male partners. In this situation, there was nothing beyond previous male partners to disclose and the strategy of partial disclosure was tantamount to total disclosure. When their relationships with women lasted for a longer period of time, the possibility existed for the men to have male partners in addition to their female partners. While the men may have disclosed their history of male partners in the *past,* they did not necessarily disclose the fact that they had male partners in the *present* as well. That is, some men disclosed their history of homosexuality in the past but concealed their current infidelity with male partners. Again, concealment could be more or less considered and deliberate:

> Rachael knew I was bisexual, she'd known for a long time, so I suppose I must have told her. She certainly knew about my male partners before I started going out with her. She didn't know that I was having sex with men while I was seeing her. I kept that quiet. What a toad I am!

Total Disclosure

The third strategy was that of total disclosure, that is, disclosure of both past and current male partners. This strategy was most commonly used by politically committed bisexual men who saw it as important in making a statement about who they were and the kind of lifestyle they wished to have. In many cases, their female partners were also bisexual and the element of homosexuality was assumed to be acceptable.

> It is assumed that you are bisexual if you go to the Bisexual Group, so nothing at all needs to be discussed although I always do. I tell women because I think it's only fair but if they have any objections then we don't get to the stage of being partners. As it happens, that has never occurred.

> She knew anyway, I didn't have to tell her anything. She is bisexual, too, so it wasn't an issue.

The success of this strategy depends on the reactions of the women themselves. In some cases, the women reacted in even very positive terms, particularly if they themselves were bisexual:

> I told my wife that I was attracted to men before I proposed to her in 1954. I'd never had sex with a man at that time but I knew I was attracted to men. I suppose I thought it would happen eventually. It didn't until 1981. It was easier to tell my wife then because she knew I had those feelings. She was very excited by it. After 30 years of marriage it added a new dimension to our relationship. She suggested a menage, it was her idea. It lasted about two years, then he couldn't take it any more.

In other cases, however, the disclosure of current male partners brought relationships with women to an end:

> Laura knew toward the end, I told her. In fact I had told her that I was attracted to men before I ever slept with a man. By that time I had met someone and I knew what I wanted. She said that she wasn't surprised. It took a lot of courage because I knew I was spelling the end of the relationship. It was a very close relationship and she didn't want it to involve anyone else.

In these cases, it is difficult to disentangle the effects of disclosure of infidelity and of homosexuality.

BISEXUALITY: PUBLIC AND PERSONAL VERSIONS

The individual's view of self has been a central analytic focus of much modern sociology and social-psychology, especially in the field of health. There are at least two important strands of analysis. First, the individual receives diverse cues from his or her society that shape personal views of self. In medical sociology, the labelling perspective draws on this tradition to emphasize the formative effects of external factors in shaping the self in areas such as mental illness and disability (Gerhardt 1989). Second, other strands of sociology emphasize instead the role of the individual in negotiating, redefining and projecting alternative views of self with some degree of autonomy from societal constraints. This strategic view of self, originating in Goffman's work (1959), also has a vital role in medical sociological analyses of individuals' responses to difficult or problematic labels (Scambler and Hopkins 1986).

These two themes have echoes in the sociology of sexuality. In particular, sexual labels such as gay or bisexual can be viewed as societal impositions that constrain the individual or as terms that may be endlessly negotiated and redefined (Weeks 1987). This duality of sexual labels is clearly found in bisexual mens' accounts of bisexuality. First, bisexual men held quite clear views of the societal meaning of the label bisexual. Their perceptions of public images and public discourse emphasized the various ways in which bisexuality was considered *problematic* by society: the public image of bisexual was seen as ill-formed and vague. To the extent that public images did have a shape, it was believed to be a negative one, particularly because bisexuality was considered very close to homosexuality. The very vagueness of public images of bisexuality was considered problematic by bisexual men. The public considered gay men as visible, well-understood, and therefore manageable, whereas bisexuality was shadowy and menacing. Particularly following the appearance of AIDS, bisexual men see their image as more dangerous in public consciousness because of their invisible and insidious potential as the bridging group, an unidentified threat as one respondent graphically expressed it.

PERSONAL SELF-IMAGE

Thus, bisexual men lived with a clearly negative societal image of themselves. By contrast, their personal views of self *with regard to their sexual behavior* were largely unproblematic. Chance or opportunity had enabled them to acknowledge and act on feelings and sexual attractions denied to most people by societal constraints. Bisexual behavior was normal, natural, and desired. Men did not consider their behavior as evidence of a pathological or abnormal self. The negative consequences of societal stigma were largely a problem for other people whose range of sexual experiences were unnecessarily limited. This is not to say that men felt bisexual *lives* were unproblematic. They could not expect sympathetic responses from other people to their bisexuality. This considerably constrains the scope for confiding and revealing personal biography to others. Above all, problems can be constantly expected in establishing and maintaining personal and sexual relationships. However, such problems are practical problems in conducting one's life, not personal problems arising from a flawed self.

One reflection of this unproblematic view of self is the absence of explanatory accounts of the causes or course of bisexuality in individuals' own lives. The search for biographical meaning is a common feature of many forms of social deviance (Taylor 1972). Individuals need to find a personally acceptable version of their past to make sense of current actions deemed deviant by others. By contrast, bisexual men in this study as in earlier ethnographic research (Blumstein and Schwartz 1977) either did not feel the need for such causal theorizing about their sexual histories or produced condensed, uncomplicated stories emphasizing continuity with a normal adolescence or chance and contingency in adulthood.

More general and most important, bisexuality was not a "master status" (Schur 1971) in terms of which all aspects of self and biography were organized and interpreted. Although half of the sample accepted the label as an accurate personal descriptor of their sexual attractions or sexual histories, the term was not often used to refer to essential aspects of their being or nature. For this reason, we have avoided referring to bisexual identity as a way of drawing together the different strands of mens' views of themselves. This would be to apply a concept—identity—which implies a more clearly defined and acknowledged view of self as distinctively bisexual than was the case for the majority of men.

The concept of sexual identity (for example, the view of one's self as gay or lesbian) is relatively recent in social history and is highly problematic as an analytic category. The view that individuals have a distinctive sexual identity emerged during the nineteenth century in medical and psychopathological literature. Such work was essentialist in its emphasis on the natural, biological emergence of sexual identity (Richardson 1983/1984). Sexology played a key role in establishing sexual categories in relation to which individuals oriented and found personal meaning. The gay liberation movement sharpened and expanded the concept of sexual identity by rejecting pathological conceptions of homosexuality; affirming a positive view of self as gay, and connecting personal identity to broader aspects of personal lifestyle, political action, and involvement in "out" gay social life. While rejecting biological and psychologistic models of homosexuality, the gay liberation movement reinforced many of the essentialist connotations of sexual identity, albeit in terms that encompassed more than sexual behavior alone (Cass 1983/1984).

Although social developments in gay sexual politics resulted in a more expanded version of sexual identity to encompass lifestyle, social affiliations, and personal politics, it is remarkable how little impact this liberalization of nineteenth-century notions of sexual identity had with regard to bisexuality. The dichotomous mode of popular thinking leaves little scope for intermediate social identities between homosexual and heterosexual. Much of the more formal, scientific discourse has also preferred to see bisexuality as either transient and fleeting, while the individual finds a more fixed sexual identity, or transitional in the case of individuals changing from one to the other sexual pole (MacDonald 1981). Furthermore, gay cultures have been particularly vehement in rejecting the notion of a distinctive bisexual identity and marginalizing men who lead bisexual lives on the grounds that such men are denying their true (gay) sexual identity and are in a sense traitors to the gay cause (Paul 1983/1984; Blumstein and Schwartz 1977). No social movement has emerged to promote bisexual identity. The social factors that facilitate such developments are complex and include geographical proximity, numbers of minority individuals, and degree of hostility from majority members of society (Weeks 1987). To some extent, bisexual men have benefitted sufficiently from gay liberation politics and have not felt compelling grounds for distinctive social and political action. For whatever reasons, there are few public, organizational, or symbolic forms around which bisexuality may cohere. Organizational and social arrangements provide external anchoring points in relation to which individual gay men may define and redefine their sexual identity, so that "coming out" is both personal discovery and public commitment. By contrast, bisexual lives have few public points of reference to stabilize essentialist conceptions of a bisexual identity.

BISEXUALITY AS INTERPERSONAL BEHAVIOR

The majority of men in this study did not describe or account for themselves and their lives in terms of a bisexual identity. Our explanation for this is that bisexuality has not yet crystallized around social arrangements that, in a sense, function to create and reproduce bisexuality as a "real" identity. Thus, for the majority of the sample, bisexual identity was not used as an explanatory construct for who the men were, as gay identity would be used for other men. Instead of emphasizing the personal and internal dilemmas of identity, the main problems were interpersonal and turned upon the related issues of information control and maintaining personal relationships. Men were concerned, especially in relation to female partners, with recurrent dilemmas of determining how much information to reveal about their sexual histories. Alternatively, if they had resolved to conceal their sexual activities, the task became the practical one of sustaining secrecy.

Information control has received a certain amount of attention from medical sociology, again largely in the context of strategies to limit the threat to personal identity from stigmatizing health problems (Schneider and Conrad 1980). Information about aspects of the body or the mind are concealed or only selectively revealed in order to maintain the individual's sense of self to himself or to others (Charmaz 1983). The objective of strategic behaviors can in this sense accurately be analyzed as protection of identity. In the case of bisexuality, the information concealed from the audience concerns sexual activities with other partners. The objective is not generally to protect the individual's sense of self, although for a few men there were concerns about being publicly associated with a deviant sexual minority. The primary objective is to retain an affectional or sexual relationship with another individual.

A number of analysts of sexuality have begun to argue that the concept of sexual identity is unavoidably contested because of its contradictory emergence from (1) biological and psychopathological work and (2) practical sexual liberation politics (Paul 1984/1985; Weeks 1987). It is also problematic because of its focus on intrapsychic aspects of personal definition and adjustment while neglecting social context (Herdt 1984/1985). Instead, it is argued that sexuality needs to be analyzed from the perspective of sexual relationships (De Cecco and Shively 1983/1984). De Cecco and Shively (1983/1984) had, like other writers, found the analysis of bisexuality particularly difficult from the perspective of identity and argued for an abandoning of essentialist approaches to sexuality. This replacement of the identity paradigm by the relationship paradigm is not intended to ignore issues of sexual identity completely but to emphasize the social and interactionist nature of sexual encounters in which identities are involved (Weeks 1987).

To a great extent, the implications of this paradigm shift remained unexplored prior to the emergence of AIDS. Now, to state the obvious, a refocusing of sexuality in terms of relationships is needed because of the central role of sexual behavior in the transmission of HIV. Much of the behavioral research has been driven by applied objectives to describe, count, and model sexual behavior for epidemiological purposes. Already, however, it is apparent that a social arithmetic of sexual acts can only be a prelude—the raw material— for a full understanding of sexual behavior in relation to the transmission of HIV infection. Similarly, it appears that the epidemiological concept of bisexual men as a distinct and stable bridging group between the homosexual and heterosexual population may be inherently misleading. A clearer understanding of sexual behavior will require the development of sociological insights into the meanings of sex for partners, and the relevance of concepts of information control, negotiation of sex, risk perception, and partner perception in this new climate. Such an agenda will "direct research interest away from the image of the sexual individual to the sexual transaction between two or more individuals" (Gagnon 1989, p. 71). The particular negotiations of sexual information that we have emphasized as central to the practical problems of bisexual lifestyle may be an instance of more general changes in sexual relations induced by AIDS. The strategic actions involved in maintaining sexual relations that we have identified point to numerous issues that can be expected to arise more generally in a safe-sex majority culture. It is an understanding of these issues which will inform effective health-education programs in relation to AIDS.

REFERENCES

Blumstein, P. and P. Schwartz. 1977. "Bisexuality: Some Social Psychological Issues." *Journal of Social Issues* 33: 30-45.

Boulton, M. and P. Weatherburn. 1990. "Literature Review on Bisexuality and HIV Transmission." Report commissioned by the Global Programme on AIDS, World Health Organisation.

Boulton, M., Z. Schramm-Evans, R. Fitzpatrick, and G. Hart. 1991. "Bisexual Men: Women, Safer Sex and HIV Infection." In *AIDS: Responses, Policy and Care.* Lewes: Falmer Press.

Cass, V. 1983/1984. "Homosexual Identity: A Concept in Need of Definition." *Journal of Homosexuality* 9: 105-126.

Charmaz, K. 1983. "Loss of Self: A Fundamental Form of Suffering in the Chronically Ill." *Sociology of Health and Illness* 5: 168-195.

Collaborative Study Group. 1989. "HIV infection in patients attending clinics for sexually transmitted diseases in England and Wales." *British Medical Journal* 298: 415-418.

De Cecco, J. and M. Shively. 1983/1984 "From Sexual Identity to Sexual Relationships: A Contextual Shift." *Journal of Homosexuality* 9: 1-26.

Department of Health and Social Security. 1987. *AIDS: Monitoring Response to the Public Education Campaign.* London: Her Majesty's Stationary Office.

Evans, B., K. McLean, S. Dawson, S. Teece, R. Bond, K. MacRae, and R. Thorp. 1989. "Trends in Sexual behavior and Risk Factors for HIV Infection Among Homosexual Men, 1984-7." *British Medical Journal* 298: 215-218.

Fitzpatrick, R., G. Hart, M. Boulton, J. McLean, J. Dawson. 1989. "Heterosexual Sexual Behavior in a Sample of Homosexually Active Men." *Genitourinary Medicine* 65: 259-262.

Fitzpatrick, R., J. McLean, M. Boulton, G. Hart, and J. Dawson. 1990. "Variations in Sexual Behavior in Gay Men." Pp 121-132 in *AIDS: Individual, Cultural, and Policy Dimensions,* editeed by P. Aggleton, P. Davies, and G. Hart. London: Falmer Press.

Gagnon, J. 1989. "Disease and Desire." *Daedalus* 118: 47-77.

Gerhardt, U. 1989. *Ideas about Illness: An Intellectual and Political History of Medical Sociology.* London: Macmillan.

Goffman, E. 1959. *The Presentation of Self in Everyday Life.* New York: Doubleday Anchor.

Herdt, G. 1984/1985. "A Comment on Cultural Attributes and Fluidity of Bisexuality." *Journal of Homosexuality* 10: 53-61.

Johnson, A., J. Wadsworth, P. Elliott, L. Prior, P. Wallace, S. Blower, N. Webb, G. Heald, D. Miller, M. Adler, and R. Anderson. 1989. "A Pilot Study of Sexual Lifestyle in a Random Sample of the Population of Great Britain." *AIDS* 3: 135-141.

MacDonald, A.P. 1981. "Bisexuality: Some Thoughts On Research and Theory." *Journal of Homosexuality* 6: 21-33.

McManus, T. and M. McEvoy. 1987. "Some Aspects of Male Homosexual behavior in the UK." *British Journal of Sexual Medicine* 20: 110-120.

Paul, J. 1983/1984. "The Bisexual Identity: An Idea Without Social Recognition." *Journal of Homosexuality* 9: 45-64.

Paul, J. 1984/1985. "Bisexuality: Reassessing Our Paradigms of Sexuality." *Journal of Homosexuality* 10: 21-34.

Richardson, D. 1983/1984. "The Dilemma of Essentiality in Homosexual Theory." *Journal of Homosexuality* 9: 79-90.

Ross, M. 1988. "Prevalence of risk factors for HIV infection in the Australian population." *The Medical Journal of Australia* 149: 362-365.

Scambler, G. and A. Hopkins. 1986. "Being Epileptic: Coming to Terms With Stigma." *Sociology of Health and Illness* 8: 26-43.

Schneider, J. and P. Conrad. 1980. "In the Closet with Illness: Epilepsy, Stigma Potential and Information Control." *Social Problems* 28: 32-44.

Schur, E. 1971. *Labeling Deviant Behavior: Its Sociological Implications*. New York: Harper & Row.

Sundet, J., I. Kvalem, P. Magnus, and L. Bakketeig. 1988. "Prevalence of Risk-Prone Sexual Behavior in the General Population of Norway." In *The Global Impact of AIDS*, edited by A. Fleming, M. Carballo, D. FitzSimons, M. Bailey, and J. Mann. New York: Alan R. Liss.

Taylor, L. 1972. "The Significance and Interpretation of Replies to Motivational Questions: The Case of Sex Offenders." *Sociology* 6: 23-39.

Weeks, J. 1987. "Questions of Identity." Pp. 31-51 in *The Cultural Construction of Sexuality*, edited by P. Caplan. London: Tavistock.

POWERLESSNESS, INVISIBILITY, AND THE LIVES OF WOMEN WITH HIV DISEASE

Rose Weitz

ABSTRACT

This paper describes the lives of women with HIV disease, drawing on both secondary sources and semistructured interviews conducted with 14 Arizona women. The data suggest that women's experiences differ from men's in many ways, ranging from being less likely to know they are at risk and finding it more difficult to obtain an accurate diagnosis, to having less access to treatment and hospice care and dying more quickly. Although some of the particular problems faced by women with HIV disease stem simply from their biological disadvantages, most of these problems stem from their gender roles and gender status, which leave them relatively powerless and invisible. Moreover, even those problems that have biological roots may be seriously aggravated by women's gender roles and status.

The Social and Behavioral Aspects of AIDS.
Advances in Medical Sociology, Volume 3, pages 101-121.
ISBN: 1-55938-439-5

INTRODUCTION

On June 5, 1981, the Centers for Disease Control (CDC) of the United States published the first official note describing the disease that would eventually be labelled AIDS. Although the first cases of AIDS were all men, within a year, doctors had also identified cases in women. Currently, women comprise 11 percent of U.S. AIDS cases diagnosed since the epidemic began—a proportion which has increased steadily over time—and 13 percent of all cases reported from May 1990 to May 1991 (Centers for Disease Control 1991, pp. 5, 8). Women probably comprise an even higher (although unknown) proportion of all persons with HIV disease.

Even these statistics underestimate the impact of the epidemic on women. Until very recently, to receive a diagnosis of AIDS, a person had to test HIV-positive and have certain specific opportunistic infections listed by the CDC (such as Kaposi's sarcoma). Scientists developed this list largely through observing the natural history of the illness in gay men. Yet women with HIV disease often develop opportunistic infections uncommon among men (Deneberg 1990; Gloeb, O'Sullivan, and Efantis 1988; Rhoads, Wright, and Redfield, and Burke 1987; Hoegsberg, Abulafia, Sedlis, Feldman, Des Jarlais, Landesman, and Minkoff 1990; Centers for Disease Control 1990). These infections may kill just as quickly, but would not result in a diagnosis of AIDS. Consequently, women who developed such infections were excluded from AIDS statistics. Only in October 1991, after considerable pressure from feminist health groups and AIDS activists, did the CDC broaden its definition to include all HIV-infected persons whose blood chemistry suggests a severely damaged immune system. Even under the narrower definition, however, women comprised half of all identified AIDS cases in Africa and parts of the Caribbean. Moreover, studies conducted in the mid-1980s in inner-city obstetric and gynecological clinics around the Uunited States found rates of HIV infection ranging from 11 to 30 percent among pregnant IV drug-users and up to 2.6 percent among non-users (Centers for Disease Control 1987); the rates undoubtedly have risen since then.

Because HIV disease was first identified among men and because most American cases continue to appear among men, the experiences of American women with this illness have been largely overlooked (see, however, Schneider [1990], Campbell [1990], and Fletcher [1990] for excellent overviews of how HIV affects women. Moreover, when observers have looked at women, they often have focused on women's role as potential sources of infection for children or men rather than on the particular experiences, needs, and problems of the women themselves (Howley 1988). To partially fill this gap in the literature, therefore, this paper describes American women's experiences of living with HIV disease.

Some of the particular problems faced by women with HIV disease stem simply from their biological disadvantages. More often, however, women's problems stem from their gender roles and gender status. Moreover, even those problems that have biological roots may be seriously aggravated by women's gender roles and status. Their roles (which they can abandon only at substantial social cost) encourage self-negating behaviors that make coping with HIV disease more difficult. At the same time, women's low gender status sometimes leads others to treat them as invisible or inconsequential. Both factors place women in positions of relative powerlessness and make living with HIV disease significantly more difficult than it would otherwise be.

METHODS

This chapter draws primarily on secondary sources as well as on semistructured interviews I conducted between 1986 and 1989 with 14 Arizona women at various stages of HIV disease (for further details, see Weitz 1991a). I also interviewed 23 men with HIV disease and use those data for comparison.

To obtain respondents, I asked both physicians who treat HIV disease and the four community AIDS organizations in Arizona to mail letters to their clients describing the study and inviting the clients to contact me about participating. I did not have access to these mailing lists and do not know how accurate the lists were or to what extent they duplicated each other. I interviewed all women who contacted me, ranging from women who were still asymptomatic to women with full-blown AIDS. The interviews, which were audiotaped and transcribed, ranged from two to five hours in length and averaged about three hours.

Half of the women, like 51 percent of women with AIDS nationally, had become infected through sharing needles. Forty-three percent of the women, in contrast to 33 percent of women with AIDS nationally, had become infected through heterosexual intercourse—two with hemophiliacs, three with drug users, and one with a husband who had received a contaminated blood transfusion. The remaining woman became infected through blood transfusions.

The women's ages ranged from 22 to 40, with the majority (57%) in their twenties, making them somewhat younger than women with AIDS both nationally and in Arizona (Centers for Disease Control 1991, p. 12; personal communication, Arizona Department of Health Services, June 1991). Seven percent were Hispanic or black, almost identical to the proportion (5%) among Arizona women with AIDS. However, it should be noted that a much higher proportion of women with HIV disease in the eastern states are black or Hispanic. In those states, women more commonly become infected directly or indirectly through intravenous drug use, which is more common there among blacks and Hispanics than among whites (Alcers 1992). Nationally, 73 percent of adult and adolescent women with AIDS are black or Hispanic (Centers for Disease Control 1991, p. 10).

LIVING WITH HIV DISEASE

Assessing One's Risk Before Diagnosis

Even before they are diagnosed, the experiences of women with HIV disease diverge from those of men. The overwhelming majority of men with HIV disease became infected as a result of homosexual or drug-using activity. Like others who are gay or use drugs, most of these men probably knew at least intellectually that they were at risk (Emmons, Joseph, Kessler, Wortman, Montgomery, and Ostrow 1986; McKusick, Horstman, and Coates 1985; Siegel 1988; Friedman, Des Jarlais, and Sotheran 1986; Ginzburg, French, Jackson, Hartsock, MacDonald, and Weiss 1986; Weitz 1991a). With this knowledge, the men could choose whether to try to protect themselves against infection. Thus knowledge could translate into power—in this case, the power to save one's own life.

In contrast, many American women with HIV disease lacked this power. Although the majority become infected through their own drug use, a significant proportion become infected through heterosexual relationships, including relationships with men who do not know or do not tell that they are at risk. Others—infected through transfusions or long-abandoned IV drug use or drug-using partners—do not belong to subcultures in which the risks of HIV infection are an acknowledged part of life. Consequently, women often lack the knowledge they need to protect themselves from infection.

This proved true among the women I interviewed, half of whom did not realize they were at risk until they were diagnosed. Two did not know that blood transfusions could transmit HIV. One did not know that intravenous needles could transmit HIV. One (married to a hemophiliac) did not know that hemophiliacs were at risk. One, who had divorced a drug-using ex-husband ten years before, had assumed she was uninfected because she had stayed healthy for so long. One did not know of her husband's affairs and one did not know of an ex-lover's drug use.

For such women, HIV infection does not seem a real threat. For example, the woman who did not know of her ex-lover's drug use was a career soldier. As such, she was required to take the HIV test yearly. When asked if she had worried about the test, she replied, "Absolutely not. In fact my girlfriend and I joked. I was not afraid one bit to go in."

Moreover, of the seven women who realized they were at risk, only the two who still used intravenous drugs at the time of diagnosis had worried about contracting HIV disease. One had discounted the possibility that a former lover with hemophilia might have infected her. She knew no other hemophiliacs and knew nothing about the devastation that HIV disease had wrought in that population. The remaining four considered their risks small because they had stopped using drugs several years earlier. They, too—no longer in touch with the drug-using community—did not realize how HIV had spread. One of these women, for example, initially went to her doctor because of a sore throat. While there, she decided to mention the lumps that had grown on her neck during the past few months. Her reactions show the extent to which she had denied that she was at risk:

> The doctor asked me if I had used drugs, and I said "Yes, I did." He then asked "Do you think we have to test you for AIDS?" And, I went, "Oh, come on." I had quit doing drugs, and I am trying to get my life together. It had been two years or three years. I just couldn't believe it.... [When they told me I had AIDS] I did not even cry. I just was like, "What are you talking about? I feel all right." I felt fine at that point. I just had these lumps that didn't hurt, that I thought was just a cyst, or something minor, because I felt great. I was [just] a little tired.

Similarly, another woman I interviewed was a former prostitute and drug user who had left the east coast three or four years earlier to enter a drug treatment program in Arizona. Describing some of her past risky behaviors, she said:

> Back east, the law is one year in jail for carrying a needle, even without any drugs. So there was (sic) lots of times when I had the money, but I would just keep using the same needle. I would sit in my bathroom 24 hours, 36 hours, trying to get into a vein. There would be blood all over the floor, the walls, the ceiling, like a horror film.

Despite this past history, when a lover asked her to get tested, she did not fear that she would test positive:

> By then I had stopped using drugs, so I thought I had gotten out just in the nick of time.... I figured I had been out here for so long, and I felt fine, I had no symptoms. I really expected it would come out negative.

Seeking a Diagnosis

Women who do not recognize that they are at risk do not have to struggle with the long months or even years of anxiety that often accompanies men's experience of HIV. In exchange, however, these women face a different anxiety, for they cannot explain their increasing infirmity once they start becoming ill.

Neither does going to a doctor necessarily diminish their anxiety, for doctors often lack the skills needed to diagnose AIDS in women or men (Weitz 1991a, pp. 62-63; Lewis, Freeman, and Corey 1987).[1] Underdiagnosis seems especially common among women, however. For example, deaths attributed to respiratory and infectious diseases approximately doubled between 1981 and 1986 among young women in New York City and Washington D.C., while remaining stable in Idaho (Norwood 1988). These figures may reflect large numbers of undiagnosed cases of HIV disease in women.

One reason doctors may miss even the most obvious cases of HIV disease in women is because they assume that it is a male disease (Verdegem, Sattler, and Boylen 1988). Research studies, medical textbooks, and media accounts have all focused on men, making the experiences of women with HIV disease all but invisible. Accounts of intravenous drug use, too, have focused to a great extent on the experiences of men. Thus, doctors may not even consider that a woman might use drugs or otherwise be at risk for HIV infection. If the women, too, either do not know or do not tell their doctors that they are at risk, a diagnosis of HIV disease may never be contemplated (Weitz 1991a, pp. 60-64).

In addition, few doctors (let alone members of the public) can recognize the particular symptoms of HIV disease in women without a lengthy and laborious process of differential diagnosis. For example, various gynecological problems, such as pelvic inflammatory disease, cervical dysplasia, and recurrent vaginal candidiasis, may signal HIV infection (Gloeb, O'Sullivan, and Efantis 1988; Rhoads, Wright, Redfield, and Burke 1987; Hoegsberg, Abulafia, Sedlis, Feldman, Des Jarlais, Landesman, and Minkoff 1990; Centers for Disease Control 1990; Schafer, Friedmann, Mielke, Schwartlander, and Koch 1991). Doctors who work with many HIV-infected patients may suspect infection in women who show recurrent and multiple gynecological problems. Yet these problems are not part of the CDC's diagnostic schema for HIV disease. Nor are they routinely described in the medical literature as symptoms of HIV disease. Consequently, most doctors would not recognize these problems as indications to test for HIV. In contrast, the symptoms of HIV infection in men have been well-publicized and are particularly well-known by doctors who specialize in treating gay men. Thus, the invisibility of women within medical literature on HIV disease coupled with social expectations regarding the kinds of behaviors in which women do or do not engage makes misdiagnosis substantially more common for women than for men. In addition, misdiagnosis is even more common among women who are pregnant, because doctors may confuse symptoms of illness, such as tiredness or nausea, with the normal consequences of pregnancy (Minkoff, DeRegt, Landesman, and Schwartz 1986). This problem is aggravated by doctors' tendency to dismiss as psychological women's complaints of physical distress (Zola 1991; Corea 1985).

Testing for HIV

While some individuals delay seeking medical care until they are quite ill, others seek to learn if they are infected even before developing symptoms. Sixty-three percent of Arizona gay and bisexual men who participated in a recent nonrandom survey had been tested for HIV antibodies (Weitz 1991b), either to relieve their anxiety, to learn if they must protect their partners, to decide whether to begin potentially helpful treatments or health regimens, or for some other reason.

The relative weight women give to potential reasons for testing, and thus their decisions about when to get tested, seem to differ significantly from men's views. Specifically, compared to the gay and bisexual men I interviewed and surveyed, the women seemed far more concerned about protecting the health of others. Whereas the men typically assumed that their partners were already at risk due to other relationships and so felt no particular obligation to protect them, the women generally believed that they were the only potential source of infection for their husbands or lovers. As a result, they felt ethically obligated to get tested to protect others or had been required by their lovers to get tested as a condition for starting or continuing a relationship.

These behaviors mesh with women and men's gender-role expectations. Women learn from an early age that they are supposed to protect and nurture others before themselves. Studies have shown that an ethic that stresses caring and developing relationships underlies many of women's actions (e.g., Gilligan 1982; Tannen 1990). In contrast, men are taught to compete rather than to cooperate in all aspects of life, including personal relationships. Thus, it is not surprising that men would display less concern than women about protecting their sexual partners.

The women were also more likely to seek early testing because they had less knowledge of the potential problems testing could cause. The men I interviewed lived in a community at risk in which the possible emotional and social dangers of the test have been widely discussed and are widely visible. In contrast, the women only learned of its dangers after they were tested. Without this knowledge, they had had no reason to avoid getting tested and had lost the ability to direct their own fate.

One woman I interviewed, for example, decided to get tested after learning that the one person she had shared needles with had AIDS. Her husband, a career military man, did not know of her drug use. Even though she suspected that she would test positive, she did not consider until too late the potential hazards of getting tested by a military doctor:

> So I called the [military] base. And there you have to see a doctor and then they order your test for you. And I just knew. I had a feeling. So I went down and had me and my son tested. He's also HIV positive, the baby. Which I didn't

know. I wish I had gone to the health department, it would have caused me a lot less trouble. Because now my husband [who was immediately informed by the doctor that she tested positive] is fighting me for custody of the kids, or says he's going to. [He had also emptied their savings account and cut off her support]. So that way it would have been all confidential. But people don't know, I didn't know.

In future years, women's experiences of HIV testing probably will diverge further from men's, as HIV testing becomes integrated into routine prenatal care. The American College of Obstetricians and Gynecologists now recommends that its members routinely run HIV tests on all patients considered at risk either because of their behaviors or because they live in areas with high rates of HIV infection (American College of Obstetricians and Gynecologists 1988). In addition, some doctors recommend, and the states of Florida and Michigan require, prenatal HIV testing for all pregnant women (Gostin 1989, p. 1625). Elsewhere, hospitals may routinely test all maternity patients for HIV infection, without necessarily first obtaining informed consent (personal communications, various maternity nurses, Phoenix, AZ 1991; Henry, Maki, and Crossley 1988).

Thus, the odds of a woman learning she is HIV-infected while still asymptomatic have increased dramatically. Moreover, because doctors conduct these tests during the course of providing other care, the women cannot hide their identity. Consequently, test results usually become part of the women's medical records. In contrast, men who are tested for HIV more often have sought medical advice specifically for this purpose and so more often can arrange to take the test anonymously.

These tests, with their potentially devastating social consequences when not anonymous, do not prevent women from becoming infected. The tests may result in earlier treatment, but (as will be discussed later) few women have access to truly useful treatments, especially if they are pregnant. It seems, then, that doctors, legislators, and hospital administrators have advised or required testing of pregnant women not so much to protect women's health as to prevent the birth of infected babies. Thus, these testing policies seem to reflect social judgments regarding women's worth rather than simply public-health considerations.

In addition, testing in the absence of any symptoms increases the potential for false or ambiguous results, both of which are especially common among women. The test most often used to identify HIV infection is the ELISA test. Initially developed to protect the nation's blood supply from HIV infection, the test was designed so that infected blood would rarely escape detection (i.e., so that there would be very few false negatives). Protecting against false positives was a lower priority. False positives are quite uncommon, but their incidence increases among populations in which infection is rare, such as women (Centers for Disease Control 1988; Listernick 1989). In addition, both false positives and ambiguous results which do not clearly indicate whether a person is infected happen most often among women who are or have been pregnant (Listernick 1989). During pregnancy, a woman's body has to learn not to reject her fetus, even though it is a "foreign" object (Wenstrom and Gall 1989). As a result, pregnant and formerly pregnant women, like persons with immune system disorders, lose some of their ability to recognize viral infections. Because of this biochemical similarity between such women and persons with immune disorders, women more often than men receive either ambiguous or false positive results. This problem, coupled with the problem of maintaining confidentiality and the serious damage that can occur if confidentiality is broken, has led Britain's Royal College of Obstetricians and Gynecologists to recommend against routine screening of pregnant women (Hudson, Howie, and Beard 1988).

Because of these problems with the ELISA test, knowledgeable doctors always run a second ELISA test following any positive or ambiguous test. If the second test is also positive, they then run the more accurate (but more expensive) Western Blot test. Even after all these tests—which can take several weeks or even months to obtain if a person must rely on the public health system—doctors may be unable to determine whether a person is infected. Women who find themselves in this situation face great difficulties in knowing how to proceed with their lives. For example, one woman I interviewed had received two positive ELISA results followed by two indeterminate Western Blot tests and then a negative ELISA. Although her doctors told her they did not think she was infected, she reported:

> I don't feel ready to go out and celebrate. I don't feel ready to accept the negative [test result] at face value, in light of everything else. So I will in two months test again. I may, depending on what the doctor recommends ... re-test sooner than that. So I don't know what that means I am right now. I don't know what my status is. I don't feel confident saying it's either or. I feel like I'm kind of in limbo.

Even those who in the end prove uninfected find their lives changed by the weeks or months they spend, in essence, as people with HIV disease. Nor does this experience necessarily end should they prove uninfected. Some find that their friends or colleagues will not trust the final test results and continue to interact with them as if they were infected. Some additionally find that they themselves cannot accept their final, negative, result. For example, the woman described above subsequently received a second negative ELISA and a third indeterminate Western Blot. At a follow-up interview, she said:

> I will probably never feel totally comfortable unless I really turn up negative on

test for the virus itself rather than for antibodies to the virus]. I'll always have
that question, that doubt. I can't ever escape it.

Moreover, she now feared discrimination from potential employers and
insurers and had been threatened by lawsuits from both a former employer
and from another individual who feared they would be stigmatized because
of their connections to her.

Seeking Knowledge Following Diagnosis

Following diagnosis, some individuals prefer to avoid learning about their
potential fate. Many others, however, decide to combat their illness actively
(Weitz 1989). They strive to learn as much as they can about HIV disease and
about how to keep it from overwhelming their lives. Through this information,
individuals can develop a sense of control over their lives and, consequently,
reduce the stress of living with this devastating illness.

This search for information is especially difficult for women. The medical
literature on HIV disease largely relies on studies conducted with gay men or,
less commonly, men who use intravenous drugs. Women remain almost
invisible in this literature, seemingly unworthy of notice. Of the 76,000 items
of educational material listed by the National AIDS Information
Clearinghouse, for example, less than one percent focus on women (Bates
1991).

Information about how to treat HIV disease in women is especially limited,
both because doctors have less experience treating women and because women
have comprised only 9.7 percent of participants in studies on experimental
treatments sponsored by the National Institute of Allergies and Infectious
Diseases (personal communication, NIAAD, July 1991).[2] At first glance, this
participation rate may seem acceptable, for it approximates the proportion of
women among U.S. AIDS cases. The proportion of women among all
Americans infected with HIV, however, is undoubtedly higher, since over time
HIV infection has spread from men to women. Moreover, even if this rate
adequately reflects the distribution of HIV-infected persons, the small number
of women participating in these studies means that doctors cannot determine
from these studies how the tested drugs will affect women. Women's bodies,
with their very different hormonal make-up, are unlikely to respond like men's
bodies to what are, on the whole, fairly toxic drugs. As a result, even once
the government approves a drug for prescription, women and their doctors
can only guess at appropriate dosages, at whether the drug will prove beneficial
or harmful for women, and at the impact of the drug on pregnant women and
on their fetuses. Women who understand the limitations of available knowledge
about these drugs and therefore decide not to take them forfeit not only any
potential physical benefits from the drugs but also the psychological benefits

they might derive from believing that they have taken active steps to fight for their lives. Those who, on the other hand, decide to take the drugs even though they understand how little doctors know experience greater anxiety than that experienced by men who take these drugs.

Nor can most women find information by turning to like-situated others, for women's experiences and needs are as invisible within grassroots community organizations as within medical institutions. Of the 12,000 community organizations to which the National AIDS Information Clearinghouse makes referrals, only 537 work primarily with women (Bates 1991). Similarly, the support groups which these organizations run are comprised primarily of men. Consequently, the knowledge developed through sharing common experiences in these groups is primarily knowledge of men's experience. Moreover, because the groups are run by and for men, their structure may reflect men's interaction styles, making it difficult for women to feel comfortable participating. As one woman reports:

> [The local AIDS organization] didn't have a support group for anybody but the gay men.... I don't hate men at all. But I think they are real tough. They think they are real tough and that we are not supposed to have our emotions. But they get real uncomfortable. I was in a group where a women was really getting emotional but the men were not allowing her to be that way. That was making me upset because I was getting emotionalized being with this woman, just listening to her. So I think it is real hard being in a group with a lot of men.

In addition, even if support groups can provide useful information, many women will not attend because they believe the groups serve primarily as gay social events, feel angry at gay men who they believe caused the epidemic, or, like many Americans, fear or dislike gay people. For example, a woman infected through IV drug use said about gays:

> They started it all. I *hate* them. I blame them for it.... I don't care what people do with themselves, [but] it disgusts me to think about it. They should've just stuck with their homosexual selves instead of passing it around to bisexual people and stuff like that.... That's why I have a hard time going over there [to the community AIDS organization] because I can't really relate to them [gays]. There is nothing we can talk about.

No support group for women has gone beyond the planning stages in Arizona, although numerous groups do exist elsewhere (personal communication, Kathleen Stoll, Center for Women Policy Studies 1991).

Seeking Treatment

Regardless of the quality of information available to them, women eventually must decide what treatments or health regimens to adopt. Once they have made these decisions, however, women often find that they lack the means to implement them. Social expectations regarding women's social worth and appropriate occupational roles condemn many women to poor-paying jobs, to less-than-equal pay in jobs that pay well for men, or to economic dependence on men or welfare; in 1987, for example, the median income was $8,101 for U.S. women but $17,752 for men (U.S. Bureau of the Census 1987, p. 449). Moreover, women with HIV disease are more likely than men to be drug users and to be nonwhites—both factors that increase the likelihood of poverty. Thus, women are more likely to lack either insurance or the money needed to pay for care out of pocket. Even those who have insurance may lack sufficient funds to pay for drugs or services that their insurance does not cover.

One woman I interviewed, for example, volunteered for a local AIDS service organization, and so knew more than most about which drugs might help her. She had not benefitted from this knowledge, however, because she could not afford the AZT and aerosolized pentamidine that she wanted. At that time, states could set their own regulations regarding the conditions under which they would provide AZT to medically indigent persons; Arizona provided AZT to any indigent person whose T-cell count dropped below 200, one-quarter the normal level.[3] Because of her work with AIDS activists (and like many gay men but few women), this woman could obtain AZT illegally from a friend who was getting the drug legally and giving away any pills that he did not need. She feared, however, that her health would suffer even greater harm if she began taking the drug and then lost her supplier. Consequently, she had decided not to do so. She was receiving no drugs for HIV infection and had stopped going to the doctor altogether because she could not pay his bills.

Children and Women's Lives

Both having and not having children can create problems for persons with HIV disease. This issue is far more salient for women than for men, however, because women are taught from childhood to find fulfillment and self-worth primarily through childrearing and because women more often than men find themselves single parents.

HIV-infected women who do not have children face grim statistics: between 20 and 50 percent of babies born to such women are born HIV-infected (American College of Obstetricians and Gynecologists 1988, p. 4). A woman whose baby is born infected may subsequently have to face both her own and her baby's illness and death. As a result, many women decide that at least for now they should not have children.

Those who decide not to have children can face substantial obstacles. Most women with HIV disease are poor at the time they become infected, and almost all become poorer as a result of their illness. As a result, they may lack the funds needed to use contraception consistently and thus may face unwanted pregnancies. Over the past ten years, however, the government has consistently reduced funding for and access to abortion, in response to a social movement whose primary goal is reinforcing traditional gender roles (Luker 1982; Ginsburg 1989). Antiabortion activists believe that they can encourage women to value childrearing in traditional families by eliminating women's other options. Currently, only 13 states provide state funds for abortions and federal funds are only available if a pregnancy is life-threatening (Alan Guttmacher Institute 1990). Given the rightward shift of the Supreme Court, access to abortion may soon become considerably more limited. Consequently, in the future, many more women may be forced to give birth to HIV-infected infants. In addition, even women who can afford to pay for abortions may not be able to obtain them. Social pressures, as well as personal beliefs, have led many doctors to stop performing abortions; as of 1988, 83 percent of all U.S. counties did not have any legal abortion provider (Alan Guttmacher Institute 1990). The extra expense of traveling to another city may be prohibitive for a poor woman already battling the economic consequences of HIV infection.

Whereas some HIV-infected women decide not to have any children, others decide to end a particular pregnancy while hoping that medical advances will allow them to carry a later pregnancy to term without infecting their babies. For many women, however, the only way to end a pregnancy is to get sterilized, for, unlike abortions, all states will pay for sterilizations (personal communication, Allan Guttmacher Institute 1991). These women must then choose between continuing an unwanted pregnancy and possibly delivering an HIV-infected baby or forfeiting the ability to have any future pregnancies. This is a devastating loss for those who believe that having children is their main purpose in life and who live in communities in which women gain status primarily through child-bearing (Dash 1989).

Even when deciding not to have children seems the only logical choice and when birth control and abortion can be obtained, this decision still can carry a heavy emotional cost. Although none of the men I interviewed mentioned their childlessness as an issue, half the childless women regarded this as a major source of grief in their life. As one young woman said:

> It's horrible, all of a sudden finding that you can't have kids....Like anything in life, I've found out as soon as somebody tells you that you can't have it, you want it really bad, you know. Children are not in my game plan anymore. And it hurts sometimes because, you know, I'm at the age where I want to have kids. And I want to go on and want to have a life.

The potential loss may seem greatest to those women (especially poor women from minority communities) for whom becoming a mother seems, realistically, their only potential source of pride and love (Dash 1989). This, coupled with the difficulties of obtaining contraception and abortion, has led many HIV-infected women to decide to give birth anyway. One major study conducted in New York City compared current and former drug users who know they are or know they are not infected and found them equally likely to get pregnant and to carry pregnancies to term (Selwyn, Carter, Schoenbaum, Robertson, Klein, and Rogers 1989). Indeed, the difficulty of obtaining an abortion may concern such women less than the pressures from health care workers to get sterilized or use contraception or abortion.

Those women who already have children face a different set of problems. On the one hand, the women may enjoy a new closeness with their children, as they discover how much they mean to each other and begin to spend more time together. For example, one woman explained how her relationship with her children had improved since learning she was HIV-positive: "Because they weren't so important [before]. The boyfriend was more important, and those types of things, and the job. And the job isn't as important anymore. Doing what I can for my children now is important because they're going to remember this." This change in perspective had also enabled her to improve her mothering skills: "I'm not near as edgy. The little things don't make a difference anymore. If you spill a glass of milk, well, big deal. Let's clean it up. Let's work together. Their education. Those things are more important to me and I'm more involved."

Although the women enjoy this new closeness with their children, they simultaneously may worry that these relationships are becoming too close, as their need for their children clashes with their growing children's natural need for independence. Difficulties can also arise when children cannot accept their mothers' illness—refusing, for example, to take over some of their mothers' chores because that would mean acknowledging that their mothers are really sick. As the illness progresses, relationships with children can suffer further, as mothers become unable to play with their children or to interact in ways the children find satisfying, especially if the children are too young to understand what is happening.

Having children also increases the stress experienced by HIV-infected women by forcing them to confront their own mortality. Many persons with HIV disease defer making wills because they do not want to acknowledge the likelihood of their own deaths. Those who have children, however, do not have that luxury, for they need to make guardianship and financial arrangements for them. In addition, although all persons with HIV disease grieve over the loss of their own future, that loss seems more concrete to those who have children. Having children gives individuals concrete images of what they will miss—seeing their children grow up, graduate, marry, or the like. As one woman said:

> My little two-year-old wants to grow up and be a garbage man. I think about it. I sit and hold him and cry and think that I won't be here to see it. And I won't be able to see him get his medical degree to be a doctor. Or, you know, what you always think of with kids.

Similarly, feelings of guilt about leaving their children behind, especially among women who worry that none of their family or friends will make good guardians, amplify women's regrets over their own deaths.

Perhaps the only burden placed on persons with HIV disease that is worse than knowing that they will leave their children orphans is knowing that they have infected their children with a deadly disease. Such knowledge can create overwhelming feelings of guilt. Although no data are available on this subject, research on the central importance of nurturing in women's lives, values, and self-images, compared to the central role of competition in men's lives, suggests that, on average, women who infect their children may suffer more than men who infect their partners. Moreover, many women are themselves diagnosed as HIV-infected in the process of getting their babies' illness diagnosed. These women must confront simultaneously the knowledge that they and their babies have a deadly illness and that they gave the illness to their babies.

Disability and Death

As their health declines, both women and men with HIV disease must find suitable nursing care, especially if, as sometimes happens, their friends and relatives abandon them. Around the country, however, persons with HIV disease face enormous difficulties in finding after-care facilities or hospices that will accept them.

These problems are especially acute for women. Compared with men, women with HIV disease, like women with other chronic illnesses, more often are abandoned by their partners once they become ill, for although women's roles encourage them to nurture others at their own expense, men's roles do not. Moreover, of the limited facilities that will accept persons with HIV disease, only a small subset will accept women; indeed, finding housing is the most commonly reported difficulty that community AIDS organizations face in helping women clients, especially those with children (personal communication, Kathleen Stoll, Center for Women Policy Studies, July 1991). Meeting the needs of women and children simply has not received the same priority as meeting the needs of men. Often, therefore, to obtain proper care for themselves, women with HIV disease must leave their children in the care of others. Thus, many women either do not receive the help they need because they will not abandon their children or receive that help but pay for it in guilt and worry about their children's welfare.

Eventually, death approaches for all persons with HIV disease. On average, however, women with HIV disease sicken and die more quickly than men (Lemp, Payne, Neal, Temelso, and Rutherford 1990). A variety of factors contribute to this differential mortality. First, because women are more likely to be poor both before and after becoming infected, they more often lack adequate housing, clothing, and nutrition. Consequently, their resistance to illness is often lower than men's. Their resistance is further lowered by the stresses of caring for themselves and, often, for ill partners and dependent children—something men are less likely to do.

Second, poverty more often keeps women than men from receiving needed health care. Most women with HIV disease must rely for health care on alread over-taxed public health care facilities. Consequently, many must endure long waits before receiving appointments for health care. Additionally, the doctors they see often have too many patients and too little time to provide the holistic care the women require. Moreover, the women may lack the necessary funds to afford the recommended treatments.

Third, although research results are contradictory, some evidence suggests that pregnancy further impairs women's health, particularly if the women lack proper food, clothing, and shelter (American College of Obstetricians and Gynecologists 1988; Landesman, Minkoff, and Willoughby 1989; Selwyn, Carter, Schoenbaum, Robertson, Klein, and Rogers 1989; Koonin, Ellerbrock, and Atrash 1989; Minkoff, DeRegt, Landesman, and Schwartz 1986; Nanda and Minkoff 1989; Wenstrom and Gall 1989). In addition, pregnant women who are HIV-infected may not receive needed treatments either because doctors confuse opportunistic infections with the normal side effects of pregnancy or because doctors will not prescribe treatments that they fear might harm the developing fetus (Minkoff 1987).

Implicit or explicit refusal to provide toxic drugs to pregnant women may become even more threatening to women's health in the near future. The last few years have witnessed an increasing tendency for obstetricians, backed by the courts, to consider fetuses their "real" patients and to consider pregnant women merely the dangerously unreliable vessels for those fetuses (Rothman 1989). These ideas reflect both the professional interests of doctors and the low social worth afforded to women as a group. This has led to such actions as involuntarily incarcerating pregnant women to keep them from using illicit drugs and forcing women to have cesarean deliveries and other procedures deemed medically necessary for the fetus (Rothman 1989). In the future, we can expect to see more cases in which doctors try to protect fetuses either by refusing to provide needed treatment to HIV-infected pregnant women or forcing treatment on such women (Amaro 1990).

Fourth, on average, HIV disease in women is recognized later than in men. Consequently, women less often can benefit from early treatment. Moreover, until the CDC broadened its definition of AIDS in late 1991, women often sickened and died from complications of HIV disease without meeting the criteria for diagnosis with AIDS. Consequently, they were ineligible for medical, social, and financial help which might have extended their lives but which the government provides only to those with AIDS.

CONCLUSIONS

Because of the particular history of HIV infection in this country, clinicians, researchers, social service providers, and others have built their responses to the epidemic on a model of disease that assumes that only men have HIV disease. Not surprisingly, this model does not fit women's experiences with HIV disease. When observers have noted that women's experiences differ from men's, observers generally have conceptualized the differences as exceptions to the model, rather than as a sign that the model needed radical restructuring.

For women's needs adequately to be met, a new model must be developed which pays equal attention to the experiences, needs, and desires of women and men, No longer should women remain invisible. Under this new model, analysts should consider any research or theory on diagnostic criteria, treatment protocols, or the natural history of HIV disease incomplete until it includes the experiences of women as well as men. Moreover, analysts must recognize that, like men's, women's biological and social responses to HIV disease vary considerably depending on their class, race, age, and so on. In addition, women's responses vary depending on their stage in the reproductive cycle. Thus researchers also must investigate how the menstrual cycle, pregnancy, and menopause affect the course of HIV disease in women.

This knowledge, once developed, must become a regular part of the medical curriculum. Because women more often than men do not know they are at risk and thus are less likely to seek out specialty care, such information must be taught in primary practice courses (which should include obstetrics and gynecology, for many women rely on these specialties for primary care).

Those who work in AIDS prevention similarly must stop viewing women solely as vectors of disease transmission and instead focus more on preventing the spread of HIV disease to women. For example, the emphasis on prenatal HIV testing, which exposes women to the dangers of routine, nonconfidential testing, would seem to reflect public-health concerns about transmission from women to infants much more than concerns about women's health. This is especially clear given the lack of any similar proposals for routine testing of men, who have higher rates of infection and thus are more likely to infect others. Similarly, many education campaigns have worked to teach prostitutes to use condoms with their clients. Although such programs may reduce the risk of prostitutes infecting clients, they will not reduce the risk of prostitutes themselves becoming infected, since prostitutes' greatest risks come from using drugs and having sex with drug-using lovers.

Finally, those who provide services to persons with HIV disease must begin designing services that will meet the needs of women as well as men. Most critically, these services must recognize the impact of children, poverty, and women's social roles on women's lives. Both health care and social services need to be restructured so that poor women who have or want children can use these services. Women should not, for example, have to choose between giving up their children or receiving needed nursing care or treatment for drug abuse. In addition, new services need to be developed that will respond to women's desires for choices in birth control and abortion.

In sum, before either the quantity or quality of life for women with HIV disease can improve significantly, we will have to develop a new conceptual framework for approaching HIV disease and a new set of priorities for responding to it. These developments cannot happen, however, in a society that continues to keep women powerless and to regard women as invisible and inconsequential. For real change to take place, therefore, women's social roles and social statuses must also change, for women with HIV disease cannot attain better life chances until women as a whole do.

NOTES

1.   The study by Lewis and colleagues is now several years old. However, it is likely that California physicians were more knowledgeable about AIDS than physicians in other states. Hence, the situation in California four years ago probably approximates that in much of the country now.

2.   Because of fears of lawsuits should an experimental drug damage fetuses, only two out of the 117 open studies will accept women who cannot provide a negative pregnancy test and agree to use birth control. The low rate of women participating in these studies is not, however, a result of researchers' unwillingness to include nonpregnant women. Women are eligible for all studies still accepting subjects and were eligible for all but 13 of the 245 that no longer accept subjects (personal communication, National Institute of Allergies and Infectious Diseases, July 1991). Few women participated in these studies because of practical barriers such as lacking access to the networks that provide information about drug trials, lacking the child care they would need to attend clinics at which experimental drugs are dispensed, and lacking transportation to those clinics (personal communication, National Institute of Allergies and Infectious Diseases, January 1991).

3.   Currently, federal rules mandate that states provide AZT to anyone with a T-cell count below 500. However, the program that pays for these drugs is funded on a year-to-year basis, and could end at any time. Moreover, no such support is available to pay for other drugs.

ACKNOWLEDGMENT

This article is based in part on Rose Weitz, *Life with AIDS* (New Brunswick, NJ: Rutgers University Press, 1991).

REFERENCES

Akers, R.L. 1992. *Drugs, Alcohol, and Society.* Belmont, CA: Wadsworth.

Alan Guttmacher Institute. 1990. "Facts in Brief: Abortion in the United States." New York.

Amaro, H. 1990. "Women's Reproductive Rights in the Age of AIDS: New Threats to Informed Choice." *The Genetic Resource* 5: 39-44.

American College of Obstetricians and Gynecologists. 1988. "Human Immune Deficiency Virus Infections." *ACOG Technical Bulletin* 123: 1-7.

Bates, R. 1991. "Foreword." P. i in S.B. Watstein and R.A. Laurich (Eds.), *Women and AIDS: A Sourcebook,* Phoenix, AZ: Oryx Press.

Campbell, C.A. 1990. "Women and AIDS." *Social Science and Medicine* 30: 407-415.

Centers for Disease Control. 1987. "Human Immunodeficiency Virus Infection in the United States: A Review of Current Knowledge." *Morbidity and Mortality Weekly Report* 36: 1-48.

_____, 1988. "Update: Serologic Testing for Antibodies to Human Immunodeficiency Virus." *Morbidity and Mortality Weekly Report* 36: 833-840,845.

_____, 1989. "Update: Acquired Immunodeficiency Syndrome Associated with Intravenous Drug Use—United States 1988." *Morbidity and Mortality Weekly Report* 38: 165-170.

_____, 1990. "Risk for Cervical Disease in HIV-infected Women—New York City." *Morbidity and Mortality Weekly Report* 39: 846-849.

_____, 1991 "HIV/AIDS Surveillance Report" (June).

Corea, G. 1985. *The Hidden Malpractice: How American Medicine Mistreats Women.* New York: Harper.

Dash, L. 1989. *When Children Want Children: The Urban Crisis of Teen-age Childbearing.* New York: William Morrow.

Deneberg, R. 1990. "Unique Aspects of HIV Infection in Women." Pp. 31-44 in *Women, AIDS, & Activism,* edited by the Act Up/NY Women & AIDS Book Group. Boston, MA: South End Press.

Emmons, C.A., J.G. Joseph, R.C. Kessler, C.B. Wortman, S.B. Montgomery, and D.G. Ostrow. 1986. "Psychosocial Predictors of Reported Behavior Change in Homosexual Men at Risk for AIDS." *Health Education Quarterly* 13: 331-345.

Fletcher, S.H. 1990. "AIDS and Women: An International Perspective." *Health Care for Women International* 11: 33-42.

Friedman, S.R., D.C. Des Jarlais, and J.L. Sotheran. 1986. "AIDS Health Education for Intravenous Drug Users." *Health Education Quarterly* 13: 383-93.

Gilligan, C. 1982. *In a Different Voice: Psychological Theory and Women's Development.* Cambridge, MA: Harvard University Press.

Ginsburg, F.D. 1989. *Contested Lives: The Abortion Debate in an American Community.* Berkeley: University of California Press.

Ginzburg, H.M., J. French, J. Jackson, P.I. Hartsock, M.G. MacDonald, and S.H. Weiss. 1986. "Health Education and Knowledge Assessment of HTLV-III Diseases Among Intravenous Drug Users." *Health Education Quarterly* 13: 373-82.

Gloeb, D.J., M.J. O'Sullivan, and J. Efantis. 1988."Human Immunodeficiency Virus Infection in Women, I: The Effects of Human Immunodeficiency Virus on Pregnancy." *American Journal of Obstetrics and Gynecology* 159: 756-761.

Gostin, L.O. 1989. "Public Health Strategies for Confronting AIDS: Legislative and Regulatory Policy in the United States." *Journal of the American Medical Association* 261: 1621-1630.

Henry, K., M. Maki, and K. Crossley. 1988. "Analysis of the Use of HIV Antibody Testing in a Minnesota Hospital." *Journal of the American Medical Association* 259: 229-232.

Hoegsberg, B., O. Abulafia, A. Sedlis, J. Feldman, D. Des Jarlais, S. Landesman, and H. Minkoff. 1990. "Sexually Transmitted Diseases and Human Immunodeficiency Virus Infection

Among Women with Pelvic Inflammatory Disease." *American Journal of Obstetrics and Gynecology* 163: 1135-1139.

Howley, N. 1988. "AIDS Conferences Biases." *Network News* (newsletter of the National Women's Health Network) 13 (5, September/October): 5.

Hudson, C.N., P.W. Howie, and R.W. Beard. 1988. "HIV Testing on All Pregnant Women." *Lancet* 1(8579): 239.

Koonin, L.M., T.V. Ellerbrock, and H.K. Atrash. 1989. "Pregnancy-Associated Deaths due to AIDS in the United States." *Journal of the American Medical Association* 261: 1306-1309.

Landesman, S.H., H.L. Minkoff, and A. Willoughby. 1989. "HIV Disease in Reproductive Age Women: A Problem of the Present." *Journal of the American Medical Association* 261: 1326-1327.

Lemp, G.F., S.F. Payne, D. Neal, T. Temelso, and G. W. Rutherford. 1990. "Survival Trends for Patients with AIDS." *Journal of the American Medical Association* 263: 402-406.

Lewis, C.E., H. E. Freeman, and C.R. Corey. 1987. "AIDS-Related Competence of California's Primary Care Physicians." *American Journal of Public Health* 77: 795-800.

Listernick, J.I. 1989. "The Case Against Mandatory Prenatal Testing for HIV." *Clinical Obstetrics and Gynecology* 32: 506-515.

Luker, K. 1982. *Abortion and the Politics of Motherhood*. Berkeley: University of California Press.

McKusick, L., W. Horstman, and T.J. Coates. 1985. "AIDS and Sexual Behavior Reported by Gay Men in San Francisco." *American Journal of Public Health* 75: 493-496.

Minkoff, H.L. 1987. "Care of Pregnant Women Infected with Human Immunodeficiency Virus." *Journal of the American Medical Association* 258: 2714-2717.

Minkoff, H.L., R.H. DeRegt, S. Landesman, R. Schwartz. 1986. "Pneumocystis Carinii Pneumonia Associated with Acquired Immunodeficiency Syndrome in Pregnancy: A Report of Three Maternal Deaths." *Obstetrics and Gynecology* 67: 284-287.

Nanda, D. and H.L. Minkoff. 1989. "HIV in Pregnancy—Transmission and Immune Effects." *Clinical Obstetrics and Gynecology* 32: 456-466.

Norwood, C. 1988. "Women and the 'Hidden' AIDS Epidemic." *Network News* (newsletter of the National Women's Health Network 13 (6, November-December) :1+.

Rhoads, J.L., D.C. Wright, R. R. Redfield, and D. S. Burke. 1987. "Chronic Vaginal Candidiasis in Women with Human Immunodeficiency Virus Infection." *Journal of the American Medical Association* 257: 3105-3107.

Rothman, B.K. 1989. *Recreating Motherhood: Ideology and Technology in a Patriarchal Society*. New York: Norton.

Schafer, A., W. Friedmann, M. Mielke, B. Schwartlander, and M.A. Koch. 1991. "The Increased Frequency of Cervical Dysplasia-Neoplasia in Women Infected with the Human Immunodeficiency Virus is Related to the Degree of Immunosuppression." *American Journal of Obstetrics and Gynecology* 164: 593-599.

Schneider, B.E. 1990. "Women and AIDS: An International Perspective." *Futures* 13 (February): 72-90.

Selwyn, P.A., R.J. Carter, E.E. Schoenbaum, V.J. Robertson, R.S. Klein, and M.F. Rogers. 1989. "Knowledge of HIV Antibody Status and Decisions to Continue or Terminate Pregnancy Among Intravenous Drug Users." *Journal of the American Medical Association* 261: 3567-3571.

Siegel, K. 1988. "Patterns of Change in Sexual Behavior Among Gay Men in New York City." *Archives of Sexual Behavior* 17: 481-97.

Tannen, D. 1990. *You Just Don't Understand: Women and Men in Conversation*. New York: Ballantine.

U.S. Bureau of the Census. 1987. *Statistical Abstract*. Washington, DC. U.S. Government Printing Office.

Verdegem, T.D., F.R. Sattler, and C.T. Boylen. 1988. "Increased Fatality from Pneumocystis Carinii Pneumonia in Women with AIDS." *Abstracts of Fourth International Conference on AIDS,* No. 7271, p. 445.

Weitz, R. 1989. "Uncertainty in the Lives of Persons with AIDS." *Journal of Health and Social Behavior* 30: 270-281.

————, 1991a. *Life with AIDS.* New Brunswick, NJ: Rutgers University Press.

————, 1991b. "Use of HIV Testing Among Gay and Bisexual Men in Arizona." *American Journal of Public Health* 81: 1212.

Wenstrom, K.D. and S.A. Gall. 1989. "HIV Infection in Women." *Obstetrics and Gynecology Clinics of North America* 16: 627-643.

Zola, I.K. 1991. "Bringing Our Bodies and Ourselves Back In: Reflections on a Past, Present, and Future 'Medical Sociology.' " *Journal of Health and Social Behavior* 32: 1-16.

OCCUPATIONAL HEALTH RISKS OF HARM REDUCTION WORK:

COMBATING AIDS AMONG INJECTION DRUG USERS

Robert S. Broadhead and Kathryn J. Fox

ABSTRACT

Although outreach workers have played a pivotal role throughout the United
States since 1987 in combating the spread of HIV among injection drug users,
there are no analyses of the occupational health risks which they must manage.
This is in stark contrast to the many studies of the risks which physicians, nurses,
and other occupations face. The analysis focuses on outreach workers' own
perceptions of the health risks they face, and how they have devised innovative
methods of managing them. The analysis examines four risk categories: physical
assault, psychological and emotional assault, work-related drug use and addiction
relapse, and demoralization and burnout. The authors' were trained as outreach
workers and deployed with several outreach teams for a year and a half in various
targeted areas within San Francisco. The field data, being ethnographic and
phenomenological, offer an analysis that differs significantly from most studies
of occupational health risks in medical sociology.

The Social and Behavioral Aspects of AIDS.
Advances in Medical Sociology, Volume 3, pages 123-142.
Copyright © 1993 by JAI Press Inc.
All Rights of reproduction in any form reserved.
ISBN: 1-55938-439-5

INTRODUCTION

Community health outreach workers—CHOWs—have been playing a crucial role in combating the spread of HIV among injection drug users (IDUs), their sexual partners, prostitutes, and other street populations throughout the United States. Since 1987, the National Institute on Drug Abuse (NIDA) (1987, 1989) has funded demonstration projects in over 60 U.S. cities to deploy indigenous workers to identify, access and teach AIDS prevention to drug users and their sexual partners in the community. As Zinberg (1989, p. 39) explained, policy and program planners have found that the mass media or drug treatment facilities cannot be relied upon to reach sufficient percentages of these at-risk populations; innovative strategies are urgently needed.

To combat HIV, CHOWs enter illicit drug scenes and neighborhoods and work directly with IDUs and other members on their own terms and turf, which typically involves walking the streets of blighted, high-crime, violence-ridden areas. In attempting to save IDUs and their associates from contracting a deadly infection, CHOWs appear to put their own health and, perhaps, their lives as well at considerable risk. The analysis explores four risk categories that concern CHOWs in conducting AIDS-prevention outreach to different at-risk groups in drug scenes: physical assault, psychological and emotional assault, work-related drug use and addiction relapse, and demoralization and burnout.

The analysis is part of a-three year, ethnographic study that began in June 1988 of a model outreach project in the San Francisco Bay area (Broadhead and Fox 1990). The findings are based on one-and-a-half years of participant observation with CHOWs at work, during which time the authors also trained as CHOWs and worked as members of different outreach teams. Broadhead joined a three-member team deployed in a large Latino community that worked primarily with street IDUs and prostitutes. Fox worked in two communities: with a three-member team involved with homeless and runaway youth who engage in various drug-and-sex trade activities; and a six-member team deployed in the city's largest adult sex trade, homeless, and drug-using zone. The analysis is based on these observations in the field, and on formal interviews with 24 of the 33 CHOWs employed by the project between July 1988 and January 1990.[1]

During the study period, the outreach-project staff consisted of an equal number of men and women. Approximately half were African-Americans, one third Latinos, one Asian, and the remainder were Caucasian. While a few of the CHOWs have considerable formal and even graduate education, and others have trade skills and extensive job experience, virtually all were hired because their backgrounds contain a special combination of conventional and street-based credentials. For example, many of the CHOWs have succeeded at converting a former drug addiction or prison record into an asset that prepares them to work with street populations in combating AIDS.

Compared to other occupations on the front lines of fighting HIV, CHOWs' efforts have received very little attention or discussion in either medical sociology or other relevant disciplines. This is particularly true in the literature on the occupational health risks which workers face in the many different AIDS prevention and treatment industries. For example, a review of the *Sociological Abstracts, Social Science Index, and the Hospital Literature Index* since 1987 finds over 50 research studies on the occupational risks of nurses, physicians, and other health professionals, as well as articles on law enforcement officials, fire fighters, school teachers, medical laundry workers and housekeeping staffs, nursing-home workers, and even funeral directors and embalmers. However, there are no articles listed on the occupational health risks which CHOWs face in their work with IDUs.

The analysis focuses on CHOWs' own perceptions of the health risks they face in the field and how they attempt to manage them. The field data, being ethnographic and phenomenological, lend themselves to an approach that differs significantly from most of the literature in medical sociology on occupational risks. First, most studies report on the risks that various occupations entail, on the different ways in which workers suffer, and to what extent. In other words, they report on the *toll* wrought by such risks to workers' health. As Nelkin and Brown's (1984, pp. 8-9) review found:

> Much of the literature on risk analysis assumes that risks can be objectively measured by estimating the extent of exposure and the probability of accident or disease. Evaluating the risk is viewed primarily as a problem of measurement, based on the judgment of scientific and medical experts.

Central to such studies is the image of the worker as a relatively powerless, frequently passive, victim. In contrast, direct ethnographic study of AIDS outreach, as an innovative form of work, reveals how CHOWs are actively sizing up what the main risks *are* in working with IDUs, which ones are *worth taking,* and in what ways.

Second, it is common in medical sociology to find sociohistorical analyses of how the social structure of labor relations, governments, corporate and industry leaders, and even medical authorities, have worked to downplay or delay the recognition of major risks which workers face, usually to the benefit of certain interests. Entire books can be organized around this theme. For example, in Rosner and Markowitz's (1987) well-known *Dying For Work,* different authors identify factors which they believe best explain the forms of official resistance by various industries in recognizing or dealing with hazards their workers faced with materials such as beryllium, lead, radium, asbestos, and cotton dust, or while working in the mining industry (see also Elling 1986; Nobel 1986; Viscus 1983). In contrast, the ethnography below is present-oriented and based on the point of view of outreach workers themselves. It examines how CHOWs manage what they see as the main risks of conducting outreach, and how sharing knowledge with one another strengthens their control over the conditions of their work.

Third, past studies of occupational health risks typically conclude by asserting how government, corporate and industry leaders, unions, and regulatory groups can and should change certain working conditions in order to minimize specific risks to workers' health. Again, this theme frequently organizes entire books, such as Bezold, Carlson, and Peck's (1986) *The Future of Work and Health*. The ethnographic data below provide insight into how CHOWs, themselves, are shaping their work in order to minimize the risks they face on the job while, at the same time, developing innovative strategies to combat the spread of HIV.

PHYSICAL ASSAULT

Many CHOWs speak of the fear they experienced early in their careers at the prospect of entering blighted, high-crime, inner-city communities and seeking out interaction with large numbers of people they did not know. Outreach projects hire individuals who are indigenous to communities based on the assumption that, given their local savvy and street backgrounds, they are aware of the main risks they will be facing, and that they already possess many of the skills necessary to protect themselves. However, many CHOWs noted ironically that, prior to being hired, they tended to avoid those very areas frequently in the past *because* of what they knew about them. As one CHOW described:

> And when they said I was going to work down there as a CHOW I said, oh no!, that is *not* where I want to be.... I considered it very violent from a ten year-old attitude that I had.

Most inner-city areas containing large concentrations of IDUs have high predatory-crime rates, and many CHOWs feel anxious about being physically assaulted working in them. On a day-to-day basis, it is not uncommon to see people involved in confrontations and shouting matches, or undercover police hassling and rousting people in various locations or making arrests. Thus, in such areas the threat of physical violence is palpable and ever-present. One CHOW emphasized that many clients are simply unpredictable:

> You may not feel at risk, but that doesn't mean you might not get "lit-up" at any moment. For example, some asshole who could be hurtin' or frustrated may come after you ccause you're a former dope fiend and now you're paid to go around and give out rubbers and condoms. Plus some people down here are crazy. You never know. You might get caught in someone else's crossfire.

CHOWs note that even the AIDS prevention materials they freely hand out can spark unexpected reactions. For example, some women CHOWs feel anxious in the beginning about dispensing condoms on the street to IDUs (who are mostly men) and teaching them about the virtues of safe sex. At the least, women risk being the recipient of lewd remarks and vulgar propositions. But clients can react in other unexpected ways, as Fox found out when she offered a bottle of bleach to a man on the street:

> This guy got right in my face and said, "Why are you asking me that? You think I'm a hype? I ain't no hype! You think I'm a hype just because I'm black!" ... He suggested that I ought to be able to tell, and that my inability was due to racism. On the other hand, I can't just go on some stereotypical image of a dope fiend.

Thus, when CHOWs were asked what was one of their most important accomplishments on the job, it came as little surprise that the following comment was typical:

> For me personally the biggest thing would be to walk through the Tenderloin by myself and not be afraid of anything. To feel very comfortable walking through the streets. That's that first thing. And, as a CHOW, being able to have people that I don't even know run up to me and ask questions, like how do I use, how do I put on a condom?

However, CHOWs note that although the potential for physical assault always exists, their fears and anxieties diminish quickly due to a number of strategies they follow in establishing themselves.

Because CHOWs interact with people who use drugs and may also engage in other illegal activities, they first work to convince community members that they are not narcs or other undercover agents. Suspicion toward strangers runs high in drug-using communities, especially toward individuals who do not mind their own business. Also, community residents have their own turf and street-based reputations to protect. They can become annoyed when outsiders move into home territories and make claims about helping people save themselves. Thus, in beginning outreach work, CHOWs describe facing the problem of establishing who they are and what they do, that they can be trusted, and that they are nonjudgmental about others' lifestyles, including their drug use or various hustles.

Foremost, the prevention materials which CHOWs hand out symbolically set the stage. The gesture of placing small bottles of bleach or condoms in drug users' hands communicates that CHOWs are trying to help them in a practical, nonmoralistic way (Broadhead 1992). The thrust of outreach is to stop or reduce the spread of HIV, not necessarily to affect clients' drug use or sexuality.

Thus, the prevention materials themselves readily communicate that CHOWs are not working to prevent people from doing what they like to do, or are determined to do anyway for whatever reason. CHOWs are trying to help people do such things more safely. Thus, clients come to see quickly that CHOWs are on their side and trying to look out for their interests. This confidence works enormously to reduce CHOWs' physical risks.

CHOWs describe other key strategies they pursue to establish themselves further. New CHOWs are introduced to a community by colleagues who are already well established. The credentials of a veteran CHOW can rub off onto rookies as they are escorted around and personally introduced to community members. Veterans vouch for rookies, and tacitly underscore that they are "cool" (i.e., that they understand the scene and can be trusted). Veterans also encourage new CHOWs to enlist some of their clients to introduce and vouch for them. Thus, as one CHOW explained:

> When I first started working the streets, when I met someone who was "in the mix," I asked him to walk with me. I always did that: "Come on, help me hand this stuff out." Thus clients helped me become known.

CHOWs note that, in establishing themselves as members of drug-using communities, albeit unusual ones, and by virtue of the street smarts they bring to the job, their demeanor in conducting outreach mirrors that of street populations. It becomes low-key and muted; proper street etiquette calls for not drawing attention to oneself. The following interactional style, as Broadhead described in his fieldnotes, is typical:

> Deno's style was real laid back. He walked slowly down the street past men standing around, leaning on cars and parking meters. Deno walked with a bottle of bleach or two in his hand, arms at his side, his palm open. He more or less flashed the bottles of bleach as we walked by. The guys, with their eyes down, checked us out and spotted the bleach; it was revealed to them almost as if it was contraband. In flashing the offer, a few said, "Hey, what's up?" Deno slowed and moved over without looking closely at anyone: "What's up? You need anything?" "Yea, bro, give me a couple." "Need some rubbers man?" "Yeah, man, thanks."

Put another way, bleach transactions frequently resemble drug deals (Broadhead et al. 1990).

Finally, CHOWs work to minimize physical risks by positioning themselves on the street such that clients will come to them. CHOWs work to be seen regularly in the neighborhoods they serve, and to sustain consistent contact. CHOWs realize that the trick to outreach is interacting with many people about sensitive issues such as AIDS, illicit drug use, and sex; but, at the same time, to mind one's own business. To do so, CHOWs structure their work on the street such that clients know where to find them, rather than vice versa. In doing so, CHOWs minimize the possibility of approaching or interrupting clients while they are "taking care of business" (Preble and Casey 1969). For example, Broadhead asked a CHOW why he walked by a small group of women who were obviously in the sex-trade industry without offering them any prevention materials (as recorded in fieldnotes):

> "They looked like they were haggling with a potential John there. That's not the time to poke your nose into something. I'll see them later. They know where I am." However, Tommy placed a couple of bottles of bleach on a ledge in the women's view. Maybe they'll pick them up.

Physical safety is a factor that CHOWs are aware of every day, but it is not generally a problematic feature of their job by virtue of the strategies they employ to minimize danger. Thus, since June, 1988, not a single CHOW in the project has been victimized, although all of the outreach workers emphasize the possibility of being innocent casualties to the violence that occurs around them virtually every day on the street.

PSYCHOLOGICAL AND EMOTIONAL ASSAULT

CHOWs' clients live in extremely deprived circumstances. In working the streets, it seems like the vast majority of clients are homeless, addicted, unhealthy, and impoverished. CHOWs speak often, and with considerable emotion, of the psychological and emotional assault they experience in witnessing the suffering and deprivation their clients experience. For example, it is often shocking to be approached by IDUs who have large, oozing ulcers eating away their hands and arms, due to bacterial infections resulting from unhygienic needle use, or drug contaminants. It is agonizing to see the many clients with AIDS who are barely subsisting, or dying, in garbage-strewn single-room-occupancy hotels without health care or much food; or clients sleeping and wasting away on city benches because they are homeless. Since the vast majority of clients lack health insurance and other resources, CHOWs frequently accompany or transport them to public hospital emergency rooms. But there they witness the frequently dehumanized, punitive reception and ill-treatment that IDUs receive by staffs of middle-class medical professionals ("Addicts on the AIDS Ward" 1989). CHOWs attempt to run interference for their clients by dealing with hostile hospital staff and bureaucratic obstacles. In doing so, CHOWs discover that the stigma from which their clients suffer often rubs off onto them, producing similar feelings of humiliation and mortification at the hands of others.

CHOWs explain that *the* most emotionally painful part of their work is facing clients who turn to them for help in dealing with serious problems—AIDS being merely one—but knowing that the only *concrete* resources they have to offer people are condoms and small bottles of bleach. Thus, as one CHOW described, "when you ask somebody to give something up [like dope], you have to fill the void or space. That's the biggest problem—not having anything to offer." CHOWs' feelings of powerlessness are especially compounded in dealing with clients who *follow* their advice and, for example, enroll in a drug maintenance or detoxification program. Upon returning to the community, clients face the same miserable social circumstances as before, and they look to CHOWs for further help. Thus, as Lawrence Ouellet (personal communication, August 1990) noted about the CHOWs in Chicago:

> Like the CHOWs you've observed, ours assist people with all manner of problems. Offering help is rewarding, but also frustrating when the limits of what's available becomes obvious. The sheer volume and magnitude of these problems further wears down our CHOWs.

CHOWs have cultivated strategies for dealing with the psychological and emotional assaults in their work. CHOWs work to reduce their exposure to disturbing situations by spending much of their time in public spaces and sticking primarily to distribution activities. Thus, for example, one CHOW reported in a staff meeting: "This week we went into the City Hotel and I want to tell you: I've never seen five floors of such absolute filth in my life like we saw there." The staff agreed that, by staying *out* of such places and handing out prevention materials to residents as they enter or leave, CHOWs can connect with and help a large number of clients without exposing themselves emotionally to jarring situations.

CHOWs also encourage one another to set limits on their involvement with clients and to stay away from case management. Thus, CHOWs become adept at referring people elsewhere. They collect insider information on programs and services, special phone numbers, who to speak to, what to say, how to circumvent restrictions and get clients in touch quickly with needed services or help. Developing skills as referral specialists helps CHOWs sustain a certain emotional distance from their clients, as well as keep their clients' problems *away* from them personally. In referring people, CHOWs shift the burden of responsibility back to their clients and to the community-based programs that are supposed to be helping them.

Lastly, the emotional and psychological risks which CHOWs face are substantially reduced by the unique orientation they hold toward their clients. Put simply, in contrast to medical personnel, social workers, drug counselors, probation/parole officers, and other conventional human-service providers,

CHOWs do not put themselves in a position which leads them to think disparagingly of their clients (see Jeffery 1979; Lipsky 1980; Mizrahi 1986).

Specifically, compared to other human-service workers, CHOWs ask almost nothing of their clients. In striving to be nonjudgmental and accepted by clients on their terms and turf, CHOWs are not determined to change or reform them substantially, as middle-class professionals and bureaucrats want to do. For example, they do not pressure clients to stop copping, using, or dealing drugs, or prostituting themselves. Nor do they expect clients to stay away from drug and other hustling scenes, or change their friends and get a job, and so on. CHOWs do not even ask or expect their clients to assume the responsibility for getting their own bleach and condoms. CHOWs feel that in combating the epidemic it is *their* responsibility to ensure that clients are well supplied with prevention materials. This is because CHOWs see their clients' problems and deprivations as so enormous that it is unreasonable to expect clients to keep themselves supplied with prevention materials day after day. As one CHOW explained:

> If it comes to having bleach and not having bleach, and you're sick, you're going to forget about AIDS and shoot anyway.... It's just that desperation does not bring out responsibility, okay.... Expecting someone to get their own bleach when they're sick would be like asking a pregnant women after six hours of labor do she want to re-read the Lamaze method.

On the other hand, CHOWs are occasionally surprised by clients who obtain bleach or condoms on their own. CHOWs see this as an impressive sign of their influence on IDUs, but not as something that they should now expect of them. Thus, as one CHOW said, after we asked him if he ever encourages clients to get their own prevention materials:

> No, I haven't. I've never done it and I've never heard of anybody doing it ... I mean, we've given them so much in regards to bleach, condoms, information, the [HIV] testing, the results, the interviews, the teen books, the 21-day detox. We've given so much, I mean, "Buy your own fucking bleach, man?" I don't think that will ever happen.

Another staff member put it somewhat more bluntly in explaining why it is unrealistic to ask clients to buy their own prevention materials:

> This may seem simple to us, but if you're a drag queen, meth-freak prostitute living in a single room at a hotel with two other people in the Tenderloin, going to the store and buying bleach ain't the simplest thing to do. And it costs 69 cents, which may be too much.

CHOWs emphasize that their main goals are for clients to accept them as having a place in their community, and to accept and use the AIDS prevention materials CHOWs freely give away in order to stop the epidemic—bleach to disinfect syringes and condoms for safe sex. CHOWs also wish to provide other basic forms of help to clients if they request it. But CHOWs' sense of their own effectiveness is undiminished if clients do not change in other ways, or do not seek CHOWs' assistance in helping themselves further. Nor do CHOWs become upset or angry at clients when they fail to pull through on some agreed-upon plan of action; for example, if they fail to keep appointments, temporarily drop out of sight, forget agreements, and so on. In fact, the opposite is true: in being nonjudgmental, CHOWs believe they need to avoid doing anything that increases their clients' sense of failure and to prevent clients from wanting to avoid them because they feel ashamed or embarrassed. Put another way, if CHOWs do work to *deny* clients anything, it is giving them any reason at all to want to avoid them, which is quite different from the moralistic, punitive attitude that clients typically receive at the local welfare office or hospital emergency room. Thus, as one CHOW described in explaining why she ignores local gossip about pimps beating on their women:

I would not be able to serve these men if I didn't like them. They could pick that up ... I mean, everybody down there is doing something fucked up. But I try to keep it in perspective. Otherwise, if I start disliking them, then eventually they'll avoid me and tell their old ladies not to talk to me anymore.

This is not to say that CHOWs are "suckers" and permit themselves to be taken advantage of. CHOWs know that many of their clients are con artists and are into "ripping and running" (Agar 1973). Thus, as one CHOW explained further, "You begin with small steps, not giant ones. And you make sure that the client meets you half way. That's important." Still, if clients fail to do even that, CHOWs work to minimize clients' sense of shame because it leads to avoidance. Thus, as another CHOW described:

There was this one guy I was working with, a big guy, who was going around with a hatchet in his back pocket. Everyone was afraid of him. But when he saw me, he shot around the corner. Here he's goin' round with a hatchet, scaring everybody, then tries to avoid me because he feels ashamed! But I brought him around.

Therefore, CHOWs' orientation to their clients, and their methods of accessing them reduce significantly the emotional and psychological assaults that appear to go with their work. In addition, CHOWs avoid setting themselves up such that they become chronically frustrated with or angry at their clients, or feel that they are ineffective because they are unable to change their clients in major ways. CHOWs ask next to nothing of clients, except that they accept and use the materials which CHOWs place in their hand for free— a gesture that clients respond to positively because they appreciate the life-saving gifts, and because the giving is free of invidious moral judgments. Beyond that, if clients change in other way due to CHOWs' urging or encouragement, CHOWs happily accept such change as further evidence of their effectiveness. Therefore, CHOWs' orientation to their clients works to create win-win situations, which significantly help CHOWs cope with the emotional and psychological assaults they otherwise face.

On the other hand, by going into communities and striving to be accepted by clients, CHOWs witness considerable suffering and deprivation, and they are powerless to do much about it. However, an important finding of this study was the many descriptions by CHOWs of clients who, because of their quiet dignity or their life-affirming faith, were inspirations to CHOWs themselves and strengthened their resolve to help them deal with such deprivations. As one CHOW emphasized, "My clients give me much more than I ever give them. That's the truth."

WORK-RELATED DRUG USE AND ADDICTION RELAPSE

A sociological distinction can be made between the risks that a given occupation forces people to face and the risks that people can choose to run by virtue of certain opportunities an occupation provides. An example of the former would be the risk that medical practitioners face of getting stuck accidentally by needles contaminated with HIV. An example of the latter would be the risk that CHOWs can choose to run, by virtue of developing trusting relationships with drug users, of copping, using, or dealing drugs themselves. Although all projects that receive federal funds must certify that their employees' workplace is drug-free, the requirement is an absurdity in the case of outreach projects. Indeed, there are several other structural features of outreach projects that make drug use a risk worth running.

In order to hire people who are streetwise and know how to handle themselves in drug-using scenes, outreach projects commonly seek prospective employees who once had a drug problem or were addicts. For example, 11 of the 33 CHOWs in the study project identified themselves as having had a drug addiction. Outreach projects hire former users in spite of substantial scientific evidence indicating that one of the most important steps people can take to become and remain abstinent is to avoid drug scenes assiduously (Biernacki 1986). As one CHOW explained:

> Being a former drug addict myself, I've worked for ten years to stay away from dope fiends, and I admit that it is hard for me to be around them if they've been fixing.

Another CHOW described the advice he got from friends about whether he should accept the outreach job:

> They said to me, "Tommy, do you really *need* to be around dope addicts again? Is that what you *want*? Do you *need* to put yourself in that situation again?"

Once on the job, CHOWs find themselves working in communities that harbor distrust toward outsiders, and they need to go to considerable lengths to convince members that they are "cool" and can be trusted. Such efforts can easily lead CHOWs to do things that may be prohibited by the project or that can lead to other kinds of trouble. For example, one CHOW agreed to take a sample of drugs to a lab and have it tested for purity in order to impress a client group. Other CHOWs have been known to hang out with clients, drink beer, shoot pool, and so on. As one CHOW recorded in his fieldnotes after running into two clients who were on their way to buy dope:

> I felt it was a good opportunity to get into the new territory, so I offered them a ride and asked if it would be o.k. to hang out with them. They replied jokingly, "Only if you buy the beer." I told them I'd buy a twelve pack of ice cold Bud Long Neck bottles when we got to Hudson street. First I gave them a ride to cop.

Additionally, CHOWs enjoy considerable autonomy in the field for long periods of time, relatively free from supervision or colleague control. Such autonomy in varying degrees is a generic feature of occupations at the street level (Lipsky 1980). Outreach workers regard autonomy as a major perquisite of their job. Once in the field, CHOWs have ample opportunity to do other things and remain virtually unaccountable.

Given the structure of their work, therefore, CHOWs are *set up* to use drugs if they choose to run the risk, because they are already *in* the drug scene, and they face relatively little chance of getting caught. Indeed, given their nonjudgmental orientation toward peoples' drug use and a job that expects them to forge trusting relationships with users, CHOWs are pushed even further.

But the ultimate incentive to use drugs comes into play when CHOWs succeed in helping their clients in some way. Specifically, CHOWs teach clients how to engage in safe sex and needle use, instead of admonishing them to "just say no" to sex or drugs. The gesture of handing out AIDS prevention materials communicates that CHOWs want clients to see them as on their side and looking out for their health interests (Broadhead et al. 1990). In response, clients quickly come to trust and confide in CHOWs. As a show of gratitude for their efforts, it is extremely common for clients to attempt to reciprocate by offering CHOWs many things: help in distributing AIDS prevention materials, introductions to new clients, access to black-market goods and services, discounts on drugs, or drugs as gifts. As one CHOW described:

> My only problem was that once I got people into detox and helped people, I was offered drugs.... People putting it in my pockets "when I wasn't looking." Like, "she wants it but she can't take it so we'll slip it in her pocket."

A main finding of the study, however, was that even with the structural incentives and the nature of the work itself, a majority of the CHOWs with the project did not use drugs and did not experience drug-related work problems. Drug use was a risk that most of the CHOWs chose not to run, or if they did, they went about it responsibly and with moderation, as the vast majority of adult drug users/drinkers do in all occupations and across all social classes (Goode 1989).

However, based on confirmed staff reports and our own first-hand observations since 1988, approximately one-third of the CHOWs had significant drug-related work problems. Many of them are no longer with the project. Such problems included patterns of not showing up for work or quitting early; erratic performance, such as missing appointments and failing to complete assignments; persistent accusations by clients and other CHOWs of dealing drugs, employing clients to distribute or sell drugs, or fencing stolen merchandise; coming to work high or drinking and using drugs on the job; and a marked deterioration in attitude toward work, the outreach project, and clients.

In addition, another important finding is that, of the 11 CHOWs who publicly identified themselves within the project as having had a drug addiction, only three experienced drug-related work problems. In contrast, of 11 CHOWs who were commonly known in the project to use drugs casually but did not identify themselves as having a problem, seven experienced drug-related problems. Most of the drug use involved alcohol and/or cocaine, but heroin was also used.

Although these findings can only be suggestive due to the small sample size, work-related drug problems appear to be much *less* of a risk for CHOWs who self-identify as former drug abusers. This is probably because many former addicts have publicly sworn off drugs and committed themselves to complete abstinence, and because they tend to be active members of support groups such as Narcotics or Alcoholics Anonymous. Thus, those who slip get immediate attention and encouragement from significant others to recommit themselves to abstinence, whereas casual drug users most certainly take drugs more often (again, including alcohol), and are disinclined to let others know that they may be having a problem. Indeed, casual users are inclined to deny that they have a problem at all, even if others tell them directly that they do and that drugs are affecting their performance on the job.

DEMORALIZATION AND BURNOUT

Some former and current CHOWs speak of burnout, but they do not list their clients or the squalor and danger they face in helping clients as factors that seriously wear them down. This is because, as revealed above, while CHOWs are unable to have an impact on these larger problems, they are very successful at being accepted and trusted by their clients. Compared to other street-level occupations, CHOWs' orientation leads them away from developing a disparaging occupational attitude toward their clients. Rather, CHOWs see the structure of the outreach project, and problems internal to it, such as their relations with other CHOWs, as the main source of their work-related stress.

With respect to other CHOWs, outreach projects rely upon hiring people who are street savvy: people who know how to handle themselves in drug and other high-risk scenes and who can understand and avoid hustles and con jobs. In hiring people with hustling experience, however, outreach projects are structurally destined to recruit some CHOWs who end up pulling con jobs on the projects themselves, or on clients and colleagues. Such misconduct by even a few CHOWs, especially if they are project veterans or occupants of higher staff positions, constitutes an important source of job-related stress that frustrates and infuriates the remaining CHOW staff.

For example, many staff members have spoken of one CHOW's drug use and dealing scheme that has gone on for years. The scheme not only disturbs many staff, but it has undermined some CHOWs' ability to become established in certain communities, as the following member explained before he left the project:

> I hate Sam, man, I just want to kill that dude. I'm just ready to say screw this job! ... And Sam, he's still dealin' on the job! He's got four guys that I know of workin' for him. And they [clients] ask me if I use, and I tell them, "No man, I don't anymore" ... The reason it bothers me is that it makes me look like a fool. I'm out there trying to do something about this epidemic. So what does Sam do? He tells the guys on the street not to say anything to me.

Another CHOW commented with a grin to Fox as they were working a street, "This job's perfect if you want to run a scam." The CHOW's observation is correct in one way: outreach work legitimizes CHOWs' close association with drug users and membership in street hustling scenes. However, when the same CHOW was later discovered trying to sell stolen merchandise to community members and then fired, his observation proved to be incorrect in another way: the entire CHOW staff makes it their business to be plugged into the underground grapevine in the communities they serve. Thus, the few CHOWs who use their job as a front are bound to be discovered by their colleagues, and quickly in most cases. In addition, the CHOW staff are well situated to discover those among them—also a minority—who abuse their job in small ways, like shopping at the mall while "in the field," or goofing off with clients, hanging out in bars drinking beer, playing pool, and getting high. The staff's discoveries of such misconduct—little acts of misconduct if they persist, and definitely big transgressions like dealing—have a strong demoralizing effect on the outreach staff as a whole.

CHOWs also experience considerable anxiety about the chronic instability of the outreach project and their jobs. The survival of the project is problematic due to uncertainties in the funding of AIDS projects generally (Krieger 1988). The project directors' frequent assurances that they are furiously writing grant proposals more often increase CHOWs' anxieties than soothes them.

But even if their positions were secure, CHOWs complain of being seriously underpaid, particularly for the unusual risks they take and the innovative nature of their work. Compared to the salaries of other street-level occupations, CHOWs' salaries are consistently lower, as the following entry-level wage comparisons reveal:[2]

Community Health Outreach Worker (CHOW)	$19,980
Animal Control Officer	$20,775
Utility Meter Reader	$22,068
Traffic Meter Officer	$22,932
Letter Carrier	$24,181
Street Sweeper	$27,744

CHOWs emphasize, however, that what is galling about their salary is not simply that it is low, given the risks and challenges they face, but that it is demeaning. On one hand, the project's success[3] rests importantly on the special street-based credentials, contacts, and skills that CHOWs bring to the project. Yet the low salary expresses structurally a devaluation and low regard for those very skills and credentials (for a similar analysis, see Diamond 1983).

On the other hand, the project directors in staff meetings often heap enormous praise on CHOWs for their special expertise and excellent work, and boast that CHOWs are the backbone of the outreach project. Certainly this praise is well deserved in light of the risks that CHOWs take. But part of the street smarts that CHOWs bring to the job is the ability to spot a con job when they see one. Thus, the project directors' enormous praise, in light of the pitiful salary they attach to each outreach position, strikes many CHOWs as hollow rhetoric and a "cooling out" tactic—perhaps a con job itself (Goffman 1952). Thus, as one said in a special staff meeting devoted to stress management:

> Don't patronize us. As it stands, we're in a position of having to work our ass off in dangerous situations and not adequately compensated. This situation leads to where your mind and attitude become compromised.

In response, just as CHOWs do not permit their clients to take advantage of them, they work to ensure that the outreach project does not either. As discussed above, the structure of outreach projects gives CHOWs considerable autonomy in the field, and CHOWs come to relish it as an important, alternative form of compensation—one that allows them to make up for other deficiencies in their job, like their salaries.

First, CHOWs structure their working hours in ways that accommodate both their clients' schedules, which vary considerably among street populations, and their own personal needs. Some CHOWs begin work in the afternoon and go well into the evening, while others work in the mornings and quit in mid-afternoon; some put in hours during weekends, or on busy holidays when many of their clients' drug use may increase. CHOWs also organize their days to accommodate personal matters, such as educational programs, artistic pursuits, avocations, and even other part-time jobs. Frankly, some CHOWs keep "banker's hours," as one of the project directors acknowledged, but then noted: "Well, we don't pay them a helluva lot, so we've got to cut them some slack." Thus, some CHOWs make their job more lucrative by making it part-time.

Second, CHOWs use their autonomy on the job to expand their positions into other "professional" activities they care about. For example, some CHOWs have strong social and political concerns. In their capacity as AIDS workers, they feel justified in devoting considerable time and energy to serving on various community-planning or interest groups, such as those working to help the homeless, lesbians and gays, minority ethnic groups, and various social action groups.

Finally, veteran CHOWs see a larger career potential for themselves as outreach experts. Their skills in conducting street-based outreach among IDUs and other street populations are rare, and some CHOWs are in demand as consultants or to provide in-service training to other projects starting up around the country. CHOWs are also called upon by newspapers or governmental panels to serve as spokespersons for drug-using and other underground populations who have little or no voice of their own. In doing so, CHOWs are developing their skills in public speaking and organizing presentations for different groups. Based on their experience in the field and their orientation to clients, CHOWs are finding that they have a unique perspective to offer. For example, a team of CHOWs gave a presentation before a group of public-health professionals and their depictions of drug users contrasted sharply with the perspectives espoused by drug-treatment personnel, health-care practitioners, and criminal-justice officials. As one CHOW described the audience's reaction:

> Some of them argued that there's no way that IDUs care about their health and can be worked with—or that society should even give a shit. Others supported

us. But in the end, we said something that got them all to be quiet and think. I told them that the bottom line for us is, first, to be nonjudgmental, and to keep all that moralistic crap to oneself. That got them because they're supposed to do that too as health workers.

In CHOWs' presentations, drug injectors are not described as unreachable and uncooperative. CHOWs speak of their success in accessing IDUs and gaining their trust. Nor are IDUs described as pathological and self-destructive. CHOWs describe their clients' concerns about contracting HIV and their desire to protect themselves. Finally, IDUs are not described as perverts and deviants who deserve arrest and punishment because they pose a threat to the community. CHOWs describe the chronic poverty and blighted environments in which their clients live, and clients' neglect or ill-treatment by local service agencies. What clients need, CHOWs argue, is substantially increased, basic assistance: help in finding shelter, food, transportation, medical and child care, and real opportunities to help themselves. In the meantime, CHOWs speak of the impressive ways in which drug users and other street populations have responded positively to their health messages and made significant strides in changing their behavior. Most audiences are taken aback at what CHOWs have to say about their clients and fighting AIDS.

On the other hand, there are some workers who do not see much of a future career doing outreach and who do not succeed in managing many of the other problems discussed above; that is, they do not succeed as CHOWs. For example, at least five of the 16 CHOWs who left the project between June 1988 and January 1990, did so for reasons suggesting work-related stress. The remaining eleven CHOWs left for a variety of reasons: another job, disagreements with the philosophy and administration of the project, personal reasons, or because they were discharged for some of the indiscretions mentioned above.

However, for those CHOWs who remained with the project (the majority) the occupational risks of demoralization and burnout had disappeared early on because of the street smarts the CHOWs brought to the project to watch their own backs, both individually and collectively, and to exploit creatively the autonomy that comes with their job working the streets.

CONCLUSION

AIDS outreach among IDUs is considered in some quarters to be a major advance in public-health intervention ("AIDS Programs" 1990). This is particularly significant because the special skills and knowledge needed to do the work are brought to projects by many persons recruited essentially from the streets. The analysis above, based on the points of view of outreach workers themselves, revealed that while it may be dangerous working on drug users' terms and turf, CHOWs have been actively sizing up the main risks, deciding which ones are worth taking and in what ways. In contrast, analyses which assume that such risks can be objectively measured by estimating probabilities of harm would entirely miss how CHOWs work to reduce their exposure to certain risks by controlling much of the interactional space within which they work.

CHOWs exercise substantial influence over determining the conditions of their work and what they experience on the job. Thus, in even the most beleaguered of circumstances, the analysis revealed that CHOWs frequently find themselves inspired by their many troubled clients, and that much of the emotional and psychological stress they ostensibly face on the job is mitigated by CHOWs suspending their own moral judgments about their clients. Indeed, CHOWs *create* stress for themselves if their orientation toward clients is anything but nonjudgmental; any other orientation simply increases their clients' problems, such as their sense of shame and failure, or their disinclination to seek out help or trust anyone.

In contrast, while CHOWs work to sustain a nonjudgmental orientation toward their clients, the larger society within which CHOWs work *is* very judgmental toward their clients, and toward *them* as well. For example, the very credentials which projects look for in hiring outreach workers are the same that often keep people from getting a good job; for example, a personal knowledge of and experience in illicit drug scenes; street smarts about hustles and con jobs, substantial experience on the street, empathy for and identification with members of the underclass, and so on. Indeed, because of such credentials, it is doubtful that project directors could write higher salaries for outreach workers into their grant proposals even if they wanted to. Thus, people who agree to work as CHOWs are put in a structural bind by society: they are asked to give in very special ways to their clients in order to help them, but there is nothing special given to CHOWs in return for the work they do. CHOWs remain at or near the bottom of the socio-occupational ladder in terms of wages and resources at their disposal. This is so even though, out of desperation and the failure of conventional expertise, society must now turn to the streets to find the special skills and expertise necessary to fight the epidemic spread of a deadly virus.

ACKNOWLEDGMENT

This research was funded by a grant from the National Institute on Drug Abuse (DA05517). A different version of the paper was presented at the Sixth International AIDS conference in San Francisco, June 1990. The authors wish to thank the entire outreach-project staff who participated in the study: outreach workers, researchers, and administrators. We wish to thank Gayle N. Williams who assisted us in the data collection, and Christine Zak-Lewis for transcribing the taped interviews. We also wish to thank the following for their thoughtful reactions to the paper: Michael Aldrich, Patricia Evans, Samuel Friedman, Peter Hartsock, Jerry Mandel, John A. Newmeyer, Lawrence Ouellett, Joyce Rivera-Beckman, Marsha Rosenbaum, Leonard Schatzman, Anselm Strauss, Dan Waldorf, Eddie Washington, John K. Watters, and the anonymous reviewers.

NOTES

1. Some of the CHOWS were interviewed during and after their tenure with the project. The names of project staff members appearing in the text are pseudonyms.

2. Based on figures given over the telephone in May 1990 by the outreach project, the United States Postal Service, Pacific Gas and Electric Company, and the San Francisco City and County Personnel Office and Department of Public Works.

3. Studies conducted in many different cities have reported impressive data bearing on the success of outreach workers in working with drug addicts. For example, John Watters' Urban Health Study in San Francisco, which has been epidemiologically tracking the AIDS epidemic among injection drug users since 1986, reports significant increases in the proportion of users who no longer share needles, and substantial increases in the use of bleach among those who still do share: "Adoption of bleach rapidly followed implementation of street outreach in mid-1986 ... major behavior change occurred immediately following the implementation of outreach and bleach distribution" (Watters et. al. 1990. pp. 3-4). In addition, a seroprevalence rate of HIV among injection drug users has held steady at 17 percent for the last three years. See also the news report from the Center for Disease Control ("AIDS Programs" 1990).

REFERENCES

"Addicts on the AIDS Ward." 1989. *San Francisco Examiner* (July 16), p. E1.

Agar, M. 1973. *Ripping and Running: A Formal Ethnography of Urban Heroin Addicts.* New York: Seminar Press.

"AIDS Programs are Successfully Enlisted in Drug Addiction Fight." 1990. *The New York Times* (August 10), p. A140.

Bezold, C., Carlson R.J. and J.C. Peck. 1986. *The Future of Work and Health.* Dover, MA: Auburn House.

Biernacki, P. 1986. *Pathways From Addiction: Recovery Without Treatment.* Philadelphia, PA: Temple University Press.

Broadhead, R.S. 1992. "Social Constructions of Bleach in Combating AIDS among Injection Drug Users." *Journal of Drug Issues* 21(4): 713-737.

Broadhead, R.S. and K.J. Fox. 1990. "Takin' It to the Streets: AIDS Outreach as Ethnography." *Journal of Contemporary Ethnography* 18 (4): 322-348.

Broadhead, R.S., K.J. Fox, and F. Espada. 1990. "AIDS Outreach Research." *Society* 27(September/October): 66-70.

Diamond. T. 1983. "Nursing Homes as Trouble." *Urban Life* 12(October): 269-286.

Elling, R.H. 1986. *The Struggle for Workers' Health: A Study of Six Industrialized Countries.* Farmingdale, NY: Baywood.

Goffman, E. 1952. "Cooling the Mark Out: Some Aspects of Adaptation to Failure." *Psychiatry* 15: 451-463.

Goode, E. 1989. *Drugs in American Society.* New York: Alfred Knopf.

Jeffery, R. 1979. "Normal Rubbish: Deviant Patients in Casualty Departments." *Sociology of Health and Illness* 1: 90-107.

Krieger, N. 1988. "AIDS Funding: Competing Needs and the Politics of Priorities." *International Journal of Health Services* 18(4): 521-541.

Lipsky, M. 1980. *Street-Level Bureaucracy: Dilemmas of the Individual in Public Services.* New York: Russell Sage Foundation.

Mizrahi, T. 1986. *Getting Rid of Patients: Contradictions in The Socialization of Physicians.* New Brunswick, NJ: Rutgers University Press.

Newmeyer, J.A. 1988. "Why bleach? Fighting AIDS Contagion among Intravenous Drug Users," *Journal of Psychoactive Drugs* 20((2): 159-164.

National Institute on Drug Abuse. 1987. AIDS community outreach demonstration project grant announcement, DA-87-13 (January).

National Institute on Drug Abuse. 1989. *NIDA's National AIDS Demonstration Research (NADR) Project.* Washington, DC: U.S. Government Printing Office.

Nelkin, D. and M.S. Brown. 1984. *Workers At Risk: Voices From The Workplace.* Chicago: University of Chicago Press.

Nobel, C. 1986. *Liberalism At Work: The Rise and Fall of OSHA.* Philadelphia, PA: Temple University Press.

Preble, E. and J.H. Casey, Jr. 1969. "Takin' Care of Business—The Heroin User's Life on the Streets." *International Journal of the Addictions* 4(1): 11-24.

Rosner, D. and G. Markowitz. 1987. *Dying For Work: Workers' Safety and Health in Twentieth-Century America.* Bloomington, IN: Indiana University Press.

Viscus, W.K. 1983, *Risk By Choice: Regulating Health and Safety in the Workplace.* Cambridge, MA: Harvard University Press.

Watters, J.K., Y. Cheng, M. Segal, J. Lorvick, P. Case, F. Taylor, and J.R. Carlson. 1990. "Epidemiology and Prevention of HIV in Heterosexual IV Drug Users in San Francisco, 1986-1989." Paper presented at the Sixth International Conference on AIDS, San Francisco, 22 June.

Watters, J.K., J.A. Newmayer, P. Biernacki, and H.W. Feldman, 1986. "Street-based AIDS Prevention for Intravenous Drug Users in San Francisco: Prospects, Options, and Obstacles." Pp. 37-43 in *Community Epidemiology Work Group Proceedings,* Vol. II. Rockville, MD: Department of Health and Human Services.

Zinberg, N.E. 1989. "Social Policy: AIDS and Intravenous Drug Use." *Daedalus* (Summer): 23-46.

ORGANIZATIONAL RESPONSE TO AIDS IN THE WORKPLACE

Judith K. Barr

ABSTRACT

A relatively undeveloped arena for responding to HIV/AIDS is the generic workplace, where transmission of HIV infection through ordinary social interaction is unlikely. However, there is potential for discrimination, benefits costs, and disruption in the work setting. Employers have been urged to respond with policies and education about HIV/AIDS in the workplace. The efforts of leadership organizations and the responses of work organizations are reviewed within a framework of diffusion of innovation to illustrate the process of adoption of workplace policies and programs.

> *There are many tests of a company's character—quality of goods and services, position in the marketplace, public reputation. I feel that the issue of AIDS in the workplace is one such test. Employees will watch; the public will watch. They want to know if American business is capable of responding effectively and compassionately.*
> —Robert D. Haas, President and Chief Executive Officer,
> Levi Strauss & Co. (Puckett and Emery 1988).

The Social and Behavioral Aspects of AIDS.
Advances in Medical Sociology, Volume 3, pages 143-164.
Copyright © 1993 by JAI Press Inc.
All Rights of reproduction in any form reserved.
ISBN: 1-55938-439-5

143

INTRODUCTION

Responding to HIV/AIDS is generally seen as a public health problem, a medical research and clinical problem, and an occupational health problem. One arena which has received attention but is still relatively undeveloped with respect to HIV/AIDS is the generic workplace, where transmission of HIV infection through ordinary social interaction is unlikely. However, HIV/AIDS raises a number of important issues in the workplace: legal issues related to discrimination; cost issues related to medical benefits and insurance, as well as time and productivity loss; prevention issues related to education and work practices; and potential disruption related to employer and coworker fears about transmission of HIV infection or grief at the loss of a friend or colleague to AIDS.

Some employers have responded by actively facing these issues, but many more have not. Both existing and newly developed organizations have promoted a workplace response to HIV/AIDS. Three types of responses are encouraged as appropriate: establish policies regarding HIV/AIDS in the workplace; provide training for supervisors/managers in responding to HIV/ AIDS; and provide HIV/AIDS education for employees.

In this paper, the history of these efforts is reviewed to answer a number of questions about the inception, evolution, and effects of organizational responses to HIV/AIDS in the workplace. The focus of analysis is the work organization/employer. What strategies are proposed for employers? Why have leadership organizations developed as they have, and why have more employers not followed the lead? What characterizes those organizations that have responded and adopted AIDS policies and programs? To answer these questions, the context of how HIV/AIDS can affect work organizations is presented first. Then, a framework for viewing the development of workplace responses to HIV/AIDS as diffusion of innovation is outlined. Next, the evidence on organizations is presented. Finally, implications for the workplace and public policy are considered.

THE WORKPLACE ENVIRONMENT

Perceived Need and Effects of HIV/AIDS

The typical response among employers has been one of denial of the need to address AIDS in the workplace. The costs of doing something, as well as the costs of doing nothing, and the legal ramifications in the work setting raise important issues for employers.

It Won't Happen Here

The prevailing view among employers with regard to HIV/AIDS has been that it does not affect them. They have seen AIDS as a disease that happens elsewhere, and if it does happen in their own "shop" they expect it will quickly go away. According to anecdotal reports, employees with AIDS have been given unlimited time off because of their illness, with the not-so-subtle message that they will not be welcomed back (although others have returned with job changes and time off as needed). The cartoon accompanying an article about HIV/AIDS in the workplace in *Business Insurance* (March 27, 1989) depicted employers hiding under a sleeping dragon labeled "AIDS" and saying, "Is it gone, yet?" An alternative view held by some employers derives from their acknowledgment of the trends in numbers of AIDS cases; as one employer said, "If it's out there, it's in here."

A national survey of over 1,500 work organizations found that 40 percent reported having an employee with AIDS; this proportion rose to two-thirds among large employers (over 2,500 employees), and was nearly 10 percent among small employers with fewer than 500 employees (Foster Higgins 1990). With new and improved treatments, persons with HIV infection and AIDS can expect to remain on the job longer and continue to work effectively. A recent study of persons with HIV-related illness in the San Francisco Bay area found that half of those with at least one symptom of HIV-related illness remained working for longer than two years (Yellin, Greenblatt, Hollander, and McMaster 1991).

Legal Concerns

Employers who favor "discriminatory actions towards AIDS-afflicted or HIV-positive employees" may be open to lawsuits (Bayless 1989). Federal laws that apply to AIDS in the workplace include: the 1964 Civil Rights Act requiring equal employment opportunity; the Occupational Health and Safety Act of 1970 mandating safe work conditions; and the 1973 Rehabilitation Act, which has been held to apply to HIV infection, forbidding discrimination against persons with a "handicap." All states have statutes consistent with this legislation, and most apply to private as well as public employees (New York Business Group on Health 1989). States such as New York and New Jersey have even stricter laws than the federal legislation.

The recent 1990 Americans with Disabilities Act (ADA) "represents a sea-change in the way that the vast majority of U.S. employers must respond to AIDS and other disabilities" (Nau 1990). HIV infection fits the definition of disability included in this legislation that requires employers to make "reasonable accommodation" to enable a qualified person to remain employed. The law specifically bars discrimination against an employee who, though not himself or herself disabled, is known to have a "relationship or association" with a qualified disabled person. The American Civil Liberties Union found that nine percent of 13,000 HIV/AIDS discrimination complaints involved caregivers or relatives of persons with HIV/AIDS (American Civil Liberties Union 1990). The potential for disruption in the workplace should a coworker become identified as HIV-positive can be inferred from surveys of knowledge and attitudes. Recent national data (Hardy 1991) show that 28 percent of Americans still believe it is somewhat or very likely that AIDS can be spread through coughing or sneezing; 23 percent of a sample of 3,400 employees fear getting AIDS from working near someone with the disease (Barr and Warshaw 1990). Other legal issues particularly relevant to the workplace are confidentiality of medical information and regulations regarding HIV testing.

Cost Concerns

Lifetime total medical-care cost of treating a person with AIDS is estimated to be $102,000 (Hellinger 1992). Cumulative direct costs are expected to total $15.2 billion by 1995. Employers bear much of these costs through health insurance benefits to employees; approximately 40 percent of hospitalized persons with AIDS in New York are paid through private insurance coverage— in large part, employer-based (Ball, Kelly, and Turner 1990). MetLife's group medical insurance claims for HIV/AIDS increased from 975 in 1985 to 6,450 in 1989, representing a ten-fold increase in costs from $10 million to $111 million (Pickett, Drewry, and Comer 1990). Additional benefits for home and hospice care and for new and experimental treatments can be expected to add to employers' health benefits costs.

In some cases where employers have sought to withhold benefits or effectively cap benefits for HIV/AIDS, rulings have disallowed such intentions (for example, *Westhoven v Lincoln Food Service Products,* Indiana Civil rights Commission, December 3, 1990). Insurers (and employers) have been required by court rulings to pay for costly treatments. For example, Empire Blue Cross and Blue Shield in New York was required to pay for a bone marrow transplant for a man with AIDS, the insurer argued that the procedure was investigational and experimental ("Empire Blue Cross" 1990). To cap their risk for high-cost claims associated with AIDS and other catastrophic cases, some companies purchase stop-loss insurance or become self-insured and lower the maximum they will pay for specified conditions.

Previous Practice

Pressure to respond to HIV/AIDS as a workplace concern may derive from outside the organization, from disruptions within the organization (for example, identification of an employee with AIDS), and from the organization's tendency to respond to other health issues affecting employees.

Other Health-Related Employee Programs

A growing body of empirical findings provides information on the types of work organizations that have adopted prevention and health-education programs for employees, a widely accepted worksite initiative. Overall, two-thirds to three-fourths of companies in various national and industry-based surveys report having at least one health promotion program, such as smoking cessation, weight reduction, exercise/fitness, hypertension control, and health-risk assessment. Size of organization (i.e., number of employees) is the most consistent variable associated with the adoption of worksite wellness and health-promotion programs (Fielding and Piserchia 1989). Even among Fortune 500 companies, the largest firms were most likely to have implemented such programs (Hollander and Lengermann 1988). Differences by industry type have also been found; utilities, transportation, and communications firms (78%) and firms in the service industry (71%) were most likely to have any health-promotion activity (Fielding and Piserchia 1989).

Norms of Corporate Social Responsibility

Traditionally, corporate social responsibility has meant concern for and interest in the wider "community" outside the corporation. For some, the focus has been the local community (e.g., support of charities and service agencies, minority hiring); for others, activities involved issues such as the environment and pollution control (Holmes 1977; Ostlund 1977). Evidence about health-promotion programs and the growing importance of health-care services in the workplace (Barr 1991) suggests that the concept of corporate social responsibility includes not only the community outside but also employees inside the firm. The increase in employee assistance programs to help with personal or work-related problems, flexible work schedule and leave policies, and work/family (dependent care) programs affirm that corporate social responsibility has expanded in areas that involve employees' personal and family lives, including HIV/AIDS (Netzer 1991). Extending this enlarged employer role to HIV/AIDS affirms the growing recognition that employee health is good for the "bottom line."

DIFFUSION OF INNOVATION: WORKPLACE RESPONSES TO HIV/AIDS

In the classical view, diffusion is the process of communication of an innovation—a set of new ideas—over time through identifiable channels throughout a social system (Rogers 1983). According to this view, the innovation-decision process moves from knowledge to persuasion, decision, implementation, and confirmation. The adoption of innovations is facilitated by the earliest advocates (innovators and opinion leaders) and early adopters who join the leadership. As an innovation becomes accepted, more adopters form the "early majority"; once the late majority has adopted the innovation, its communication throughout the social system is nearly complete, except for some laggards.

The diffusion-of-innovation perspective was selected here because of the fear and uncertainty surrounding the occurrence of HIV/AIDS in the workplace and the newness for employers of dealing with a health concern associated with sexual behavior. In this paper, the innovation is a response to HIV/AIDS in the workplace, exemplified by strategies that include policies and education programs. Employers may decide to incorporate HIV/AIDS into existing policies (e.g., flexible schedules and health plan benefits), to adopt a specific policy regarding HIV/AIDS, or to have no policy. Components of a policy include: providing benefits to persons with HIV/AIDS as with any other serious or life-threatening illness; confidentiality of employee medical information; compliance with laws and regulations, especially regarding nondiscrimination; top management support; and provision of education for employees (Citizen's Commission on AIDS for New York City and Northern New Jersey 1988).

Education may be targeted at managers/supervisors and/or at all employees. A variety of educational strategies is available, ranging from distribution of literature on HIV/AIDS (in a company newsletter, on bulletin boards, in a health education library) to comprehensive programs featuring a video/film presentation, a health expert to explain and answer questions, print materials, and back-up counseling and referral (Barr and Warshaw 1990). Such programs can be one-time or part of an ongoing series, and attendance can be voluntary or mandatory, that is, given on company time with all employees expected to attend.

Applying the model of the diffusion of innovation to organizations directs attention to the normative context that may facilitate the stages of this process, the way organizations learn about the innovation, and the characteristics of the innovation and of decision-making organizations that adopt it (Rogers 1983). The innovation-decision process provides a framework to view workplace responses to HIV/AIDS; two major issues are addressed in this paper:

1. the knowledge and persuasion stages of the innovation model: the development, evolution, and activities of leadership organizations that communicate the innovation and that act as opinion leaders to promote employer awareness and encourage the adoption of HIV/AIDS policies and programs; and
2. the adoption (i.e., decision) and implementation stages: the type and experience of organizations that have implemented HIV/AIDS policies and programs in the workplace.

LEADERSHIP AND LEARNING ABOUT AIDS

Leadership organizations have emerged to provide information to employers, promote knowledge and awareness about AIDS and its impact on the workplace, and encourage employers to address HIV/AIDS in the workplace. These organizations have acted as opinion leaders and as communicators and disseminators of information about HIV/AIDS. Their activities serve several purposes: to make employers aware of their own self-interests in addressing AIDS in the workplace; to persuade employers to develop workplace policies and programs appropriate for their own workforces; to guide employers in ways of responding, lead them to resources, and present options that fit different industries and workforces; to provide materials and services for employers and employees, such as AIDS education and training; and to serve as a conduit to connect people and organizations, facilitating these activities. The leadership organizations selected for review represent diverse constitutencies and sponsorship: coalitions of private corporations; labor unions; federal, state, and local governments; and voluntary service organizations[1].

Private Sector Initiatives: Opinion Leaders

A number of coalitions around the country have functioned as opinion leaders to focus attention on HIV/AIDS in the workplace, provide information to employers, mobilize corporate leadership, and encourage workplace activity. The organizations described are among the most active and are recognized by others as leaders, as indicated by the scope of membership, publication and dissemination of information, and collaboration with other organizations.

New York Business Group on Health (NYBGH)

Organized in 1980 to address health issues affecting employees and their dependents, this employer-based coalition was one of the earliest existing organizations to recognize the potential impact of AIDS in the workplace. NYBGH cosponsored a 1985 Forum on "AIDS and the Employer" in New York City to provide information on how to deal with HIV-infected employees, handle fears of coworkers, and manage the costs of AIDS. The resulting publication (Warshaw 1986) outlined issues for employers, provided policy guidance and resource information, and made recommendations for addressing HIV/AIDS in the workplace. Subsequent conferences (most recently in Fall 1992) and publications have continued to probe the issues facing employers and encourage effective responses. NYBGH conducted the first large-scale survey of employees to assess their reactions to AIDS education in the workplace. The findings show that employees value workplace education, especially comprehensive programs that include discussions with health experts and that are compulsory so there is no stigma to attending (Barr and Warshaw 1990; Barr, Waring, and Warshaw 1991). These results have been disseminated to employers to encourage them to offer AIDS education and to help them design program components appropriate for their workforce. In December 1992, NYBGH received the Assistant Secretary of Health's award in recognition of its efforts to sensitize and encourage employers to respond to AIDS.

National Leadership Coalition on AIDS (NLCOA)

Established early in 1987 in Washington, D.C., to encourage and lead a collective effort in the private sector, the NLCOA represents a national membership of nearly 200 major corporations, labor unions, and other organizations. Through national conferences, publications, and an active Workplace Resource Center that responds to employer requests for information (over 475,000 copies of its risk prevention brochure have been disseminated), the Coalition has mobilized corporate leadership to meet the challenges of HIV/AIDS. Its CEO project has enlisted nearly 100 CEOs across the country, committed to "be a visible leadership example for others" (National Leadership Coalition on AIDS 1990a). The recently published guide for small businesses about HIV/AIDS (1990b) was completed as part of a five-year grant from the Centers for Disease Control (CDC) to target minority and small businesses that lack an infrastructure to respond to HIV/AIDS. In developing strategies for reaching such employers, NLCOA is working with trade associations (e.g., manufacturers, funeral directors) comprised of small businesses as members (personal communication, R. Brannigan, Director, Workplace Resource Center, National Leadership Coalition on AIDS, 1991).[2] NLCOA continues to provide active leadership to guide and facilitate employers' responses to HIV/AIDS.

New England Corporate Consortium for AIDS Education

In promoting a positive response to HIV/AIDS in the workplace, this consortium of nine corporate leaders developed a video, "Living and Working with AIDS," accompanied by a supervisor's manual, corporate planning guide, and employees' guide in 1988. Now in its fourth year, the Consortium meets monthly to implement its business plan for each year. Beginning with workplace education to diminish employee fears, efforts have expanded out to the families of employees and the larger community, including minority issues. The Consortium has endorsed and distributed workplace principles; collaborated with the AIDS ACTION Committee of Massachusetts, a major AIDS service organization, to encourage a proactive employer response; and held annual leadership forums to focus on the role of business leaders (personal communication, P.A. Ross, Manager, AIDS Program Office, Digital Equipment Corp., 1991). This is the only continuous corporate group committed to the sole focus of HIV/AIDS in the workplace.

Business Leadership Task Force of the Bay Area

Composed of senior-level management from 14 major corporations in the San Francisco Bay area, the Task Force put AIDS on its agenda in 1985 (personal communication, A.R. Emery, consultant, 1991). The intention was to develop a rational approach to AIDS in the workplace, raise the awareness of top-level business leaders, and encourage worksite AIDS education. Seven companies underwrote the publication of a manual on AIDS in the workplace by the San Francisco AIDS Foundation (SFAF) in 1986 and sponsored a 1986 conference for corporate management to encourage and motivate them to implement policies and education programs. The Task Force continued to support the development and updating of materials by SFAF for several years until it disbanded. Some of the founding corporations continue to fund leadership activities.

Philadelphia Commission on AIDS (PCOA)

Established in mid-1987 by The Pew Charitable Trusts to address the impact of AIDS in the Philadelphia area, PCOA represented business, education, health care, religion, labor, and government. The Commission sponsored a conference on AIDS in the workplace and endorsed "Ten Principles for the Philadelphia Workplace" (based on the principles established by the Citizen's Commission on AIDS for New York City and Northern New Jersey 1988). PCOA undertook a study of the impact of AIDS on the workplace in the five-county Delaware Valley area, supported by the CIGNA Foundation with the cooperation of Temple University Institute for Survey Research and the Greater Philadelphia Chamber of Commerce, and published and disseminated the results (Mattlin 1988). However, it has now ceased to function.

Citizen's Commission on AIDS for New York and Northern New Jersey

Established in July 1987 by a group of 17 private foundations, the Commission (1987) has supported community-based organizations and workplace initiatives in its major goals: caring for people with HIV/AIDS, prevention and education, and eliminating discrimination in social interaction and benefits. Seeking to stimulate corporate and private sector leadership, the Commission (1988) developed a statement of "Ten Principles for the Workplace" as a guide to implementing policies and education programs. Nearly 600 organizations have formally endorsed the principles, and thousands more have received copies. In addition to publishing reports alerting employers to the issues and ways of responding, the Commission spearheaded a Conference for Business and Community Leaders in New Jersey in 1990. With its initial mandate completed, the Commission ended work in March 1991; some of its dissemination activities are being carried on by other organizations.

American Foundation for AIDS Research (AmFAR)

This broad-based AIDS research and funding organization published a workplace manual in 1988 to guide employers responding to AIDS. Financial support for this workplace initiative was provided by the insurance industry and corporate sponsors. The manual has been distributed to more than 50,000 American companies. However, AmFAR's major efforts have not been directed to AIDS in the workplace.

Labor Organizations: Mobilizing for Employees

Union activity regarding HIV/AIDS is directed primarily to workers, but the unions have also acted to influence employers by providing them with information to disseminate to their employees, developing policies protecting employees from occupational exposure to HIV and from discrimination if they are infected, and promoting responsiveness among employers through direct collaboration. According to a study of union activity in New Jersey (Landsbergis, Caplan, and Greenberg 1991), over one-fourth of the 55 responding unions had or were developing an AIDS policy, and the same proportion had conducted AIDS education for their members. Efforts to promote a workplace response to HIV/AIDS include a collective project by three large unions (Service Employees International Union, American Federation of State, County and Municipal Employees, and the national AFL-CIO), funded in part by the Centers for Disease Control, to develop educational materials for workers in a wide range of industries.

Seafarer's International Union

Staff of this 15,000-member merchant seaman's union have offered AIDS education to trainees and other students in the seamanship school for over four years. The union's leadership role is exemplified by two activities: an education program developed to share with interested companies; and a policy advisory booklet on HIV/AIDS in the maritime workplace published by the union and maritime employers.

Service Employees International Union (SEIU)

This union has taken a lead in providing educational materials for workers and employers in service industries. A comprehensive guide, first published in 1986 with funding from the U.S. Occupational Safety and Health Administration, has been widely distributed to employees and workplaces. The booklet gives basic information about AIDS and HIV transmission as well as guidelines for precautions and infection-control procedures for health-care and other service workers. With a grant from the Robert Wood Johnson Foundation, SEIU is establishing regional offices to provide AIDS education outreach to its nearly one million members.

United Auto Workers-General Motors (UAW-GM)

Begun in 1987, this union/employer collaboration has produced educational materials for UAW-GM workers, including an informative brochure (UAW-GM Human Resource Center 1988a) that deals with facts about HIV/AIDS, resource and benefit information, and issues related to coworkers with AIDS or HIV infection. In a jointly sponsored mailing, the booklet was sent to 500,000 GM employees. Based on the workforce composition, recent initiatives have focused on the children of employees, reaching the parents through teaching their children about HIV/AIDS. UAW-GM has also developed videotapes on medical aspects of AIDS, HIV testing, and legal considerations (UAW-GM Human Resource Center 1988b). This joint union/management activity has become a model for other such collaborative efforts.

Government Initiatives: Encouraging Employers

A number of states have not only addressed legal ramifications and other problems related to HIV/AIDS, but also recognized HIV/AIDS as a workplace issue and sought to direct employers' attention to it.

New York State

One of the most visible activities was a conference, "AIDS in the Workplace: Facing the Challenge," held in September 1989. The Governor's Office of Employee Relations developed the conference along with other state agencies, Rockefeller College, labor unions, and private industry. Nearly 500 representatives from around the state attended the two-day program that focused on legal issues, education, and other concerns. It ended with a "Call to Action" from the Governor's office to address these issues in the workplace. The State AIDS Institute has developed workplace training programs. The New York City Department of Health AIDS Training Institute also provides a series of workplace training programs, including basic AIDS information and manager training.

Florida

The State of Florida, its Department of Health and Rehabilitative Services, and Florida State University Center for Employment Relations and Law have developed an extensive guide to help employers manage AIDS in the workplace (McHugh 1989). Topics include workplace education, legal liability, management initiatives, safety protocols, testing, confidentiality, and policy development. The guide has been distributed to large employers, small-business owners, store managers, department heads, supervisors, boards of directors, and public officials, for information, training, and as a guide to management.

Federal Centers for Disease Control (CDC)

This agency has been at the core of the AIDS epidemic since it began, most prominently in its surveillance activities and research. In recent years, CDC has devoted more resources to public education and, particularly, to AIDS education in the workplace. The National AIDS Clearinghouse (NAC), begun in 1987, has assembled a database of information about AIDS in the workplace and recently published a resource guide for workers, managers, and employers in collaboration with the National Leadership Coalition on AIDS (1990). This extensive directory contains about 200 items (from the 6,000 item database) intended to assist employers and managers in developing workplace AIDS education programs and in designing policies to protect workers from occupational exposure and discrimination. CDC has worked to disseminate these materials and has funded special projects and supported conferences aimed at promoting AIDS education in the workplace. On World AIDS Day, December 1, 1992, CDC launched its "Business Responds to AIDS" program to focus national attention on the need for policies, supervisor training, and employer education.

Service Organizations: Activating the Workplace

Providing accurate information about the transmission and prevention of HIV/AIDS has been a focus of several service organizations that have directed their efforts not only to specific communities where the risk of transmission is greater but also to the workplace where the "message" is both knowledge and understanding.

San Franscisco AIDS Foundation (SFAF)

Established in the early 1980s to respond to the crisis presented by AIDS, SFAF has been involved in providing AIDS education not only to the gay community (Bayer 1989), but also in workplaces. Allied with the business community since its early years (personal communication, A.R. Emery 1991), SFAF has developed materials for use in workplace education and training, including a videotape series and a brochure guide for employees. SFAF consultants have assisted numerous companies of all sizes with crisis intervention, policy development, training resource people, and implementing AIDS education programs. In promoting ways that employers can respond to AIDS, their materials have been updated to address the "second decade" of AIDS in the workplace (Emery 1990b) involving diverse workforces. Funding for this project came from 15 corporations, and over 60 business and community leaders served as advisors. SFAF's current focus is primarily on education, for example, developing guidelines and resource materials on HIV/AIDS for small businesses.

Gay Men's Health Crisis (GMHC)

Concerned about the impact of AIDS, especially on the gay community, GMHC has been a leader in developing and providing services for people with HIV/AIDS in New York City since its founding in 1982. GMHC's education department conducts workplace training programs, provides materials for employees and employers, and advises on policy development. Recently, GMHC, in collaboration with the New York Business Group on Health, conducted a study of New York area employers to determine responses to HIV/AIDS in the workplace and motivations and barriers to establishing policies and implementing education programs (Miller, Barr, Humes, Warshaw, and Reinfeld 1990).

American Red Cross (ARC)

Probably the largest existing service organization focusing on HIV/AIDS in the workplace,[3] ARC has a national network of over 1,500 chapters providing education to employers and employees. ARC has developed informational materials, including brochures and videotapes, for distribution in the workplace. The organization recently completed a national survey of 1,000 small businesses to determine the barriers they report to educating their employees about AIDS (Gurvitch and Randolph 1992).

ADOPTION AND IMPLEMENTATION OF AIDS POLICIES AND PROGRAMS

To what extent have these leadership organizations—whether they are private-sector coalitions attempting to persuade their peers to undertake AIDS education, unions helping to mobilize employers by educating their employees, government agencies focusing employers' attention on HIV/AIDS, or service organizations providing information and assistance to employers in developing a response to AIDS in the workplace—succeeded in reaching employers and convincing them to "face the challenge"?

Characteristics of Companies with Workplace Responses

Several industry surveys have focused on the types of organizations that have HIV/AIDS policies and programs. Although sample selection and composition vary, the findings are highly consistent (Mattlin 1988; *Fortune Magazine* and Allstate Insurance 1988; Business Roundtable 1989; Miller et al. 1990). Companies that have experienced an employee with AIDS are more likely to have formulated a response. For example, in a recent survey 47 percent of companies reporting an employment situation involving HIV infection or

AIDS had implemented an AIDS awareness program for employees, compared to 25 percent of companies without such experience (American Management Association 1991).

The extent of adoption and implementation of AIDS policies and programs varies because the surveys differ in the number, geographic base, and size of the organizations studied. Survey estimates range from two-thirds of large firms to 17 percent of small firms distributing materials and from one-half to 10 percent sponsoring AIDS education programs. Educational activities, predominantly handing out written materials, are more prevalent than policies relating to HIV/AIDS. Except among the largest companies (Business Roundtable 1989), specific written policies about HIV/AIDS are reported less frequently than unwritten policies that may be part of broader employee policies, for example, regarding work schedules and sick leave.

One study that related prior experience to the adoption of AIDS programs and policies found that the presence of health care and health-education programs was associated with formal response to HIV/AIDS in the workplace (Miller et al. 1990). About half the respondents offered employee assistance programs and emergency medical services; over half offered wellness programs such as smoking cessation, weight reduction, and blood pressure screening. Those companies were significantly more likely to provide AIDS training for managers and supervisors and to provide AIDS education for employees or have an AIDS policy. There is some evidence to suggest that different industries—for example, health care and human services—may have been more responsive to HIV/AIDS in the workplace (Miller et al. 1990; American Management Association 1991).

Barriers to the Adoption of AIDS Policies and Programs

Major barriers appear to be programming costs and the small size of an organization (Mattlin 1988; Miller et al. 1990). Other obstacles include lack of time and concern that employees may incorrectly perceive there is a problem. Employers responding to the *Fortune Magazine* and Allstate Insurance (1988) study indicated that three-fourths would get more involved if an employee had AIDS, if medical insurance costs went up, if employee morale went down, or if the employees "pushed" for it. A major barrier continues to be a head-in-the-sand philosophy, which may be overcome only by reaction to an AIDS case in the workplace or by the commitment of top executives (Both 1989).

Willingness to Adopt and Desire for Information

Despite the barriers, employers do want to do and know more about AIDS. In the Philadelphia study (Mattlin 1988), one-third of the companies that did not sponsor AIDS education in the workplace said they would like to initiate a program, and four-fifths reported that they would undertake one of the "passive" education strategies (e.g., distribution of pamphlets or memos about AIDS). Moreover, in an open-ended question, about 60 percent said they wanted more information about AIDS and HIV transmission. In the New York study (Miller et al. 1990), two-fifths of those who had not implemented AIDS education said they would be willing to distribute literature, and 35 percent would put materials on a bulletin board, both passive activities. Fewer would use a videotape (29 %) or would have a speaker (20 %).

The Experience of Workplace AIDS Programs: Early Adopters

A number of companies have been pacesetters, taking the lead in early adoption of workplace policies and programs relating to HIV/AIDS and supporting or acting as opinion leaders to persuade others to follow. Three selected examples are described, and several other leading companies are noted.

Pacific Bell

The need to address AIDS was recognized in 1984 when employees of this telecommunications company were balking at doing repair work in areas of San Francisco and health-care settings where people with AIDS lived and were treated (Kirp 1989). The company developed programs to assist infected employees, help coworkers of an infected employee, and educate others who thought it did not concern them. Activities included: a videotape to present facts about HIV transmission and lack of risk in the workplace; sessions to answer employees' questions; materials with telephone numbers for additional information and referral; and counseling and support groups for employees. As a member of the Business Leadership Task Force, Pacific Bell supported the production of the San Francisco AIDS Foundation video, disseminated to employers for use in their own worksites. Despite being an "unlikely innovator" (Kirp 1989), the company has maintained high visibility in supporting other workplace AIDS education efforts and encouraging employers to respond.

American Telephone & Telegraph (AT&T)

AT&T was confronted with AIDS in 1984 when their "largest union threatened a walkout after an employee with AIDS returned to work (Gallagher 1988). It quickly became clear that AIDS education was needed to allay fears, inform employees of the facts about AIDS, and change behaviors that could result in transmission of HIV infection. The AIDS education program includes a videotape and discussion with a health professional; articles in the employee newsletter and other communications; and referral to resources for additional information. AIDS prevention is integrated into "Total Life

Concept," the health education program. AT&T has no separate policy on AIDS; rather AIDS is treated as any life-threatening illness, and infected workers are accommodated in their jobs so that they can continue to work as long as possible. AT&T has supported the San Francisco AIDS Foundation and talked about its own experience and policy in an effort to encourage other employers to directly address AIDS in the workplace.

International Business Machines (IBM) Corporation

IBM's AIDS policy, developed in 1985, established five elements: no testing of employees for AIDS; confidentiality of employees with AIDS; full health benefits including long-term disability; job accommodations to keep employees at work as long as possible; and providing AIDS information and education. The education program includes an AIDS video available through the IBM Employee Video Library (for viewing at home with family); an AIDS education booklet mailed to each employee; management newsletter articles and bulletin board notices; information, counseling, and referral provided through the medical department and employee assistance program; presentations for employees including question and answer session with a medical professional; and ongoing management training. IBM has made contributions to AIDS research and service organizations and loaned executives to help promote and carry out workplace education activities, for example, at the National Leadership Coalition on AIDS. These activities have the expressed intention of safeguarding employees and demonstrating corporate leadership in dealing with AIDS (Haughie 1987).

Other Early Adopters: 1984-1985

Levi-Strauss had the first corporate AIDS program and has remained a prime leader. Its President, Robert Haas, was the major innovator who put AIDS on the agenda of the Business Leadership Task Force and continues to be a strong business spokesperson promoting workplace AIDS education nationally (personal communication, A.R. Emery, 1991). The company has provided financial support for numerous AIDS efforts, including programs to assess the needs of small businesses related to HIV/AIDS and to develop guidelines and programs for small business HIV/AIDS activities (personal communication, R. Brannigan 1991).

Wells Fargo Bank was one of the first employers to survey its employees to determine their knowledge and attitudes about AIDS; the company was an early supporter of the Business Leadership Task Force.

Early Adopters: 1986-1987

Digital Equipment Corporation, a founding member of the New England Consortium on AIDS, has developed a proactive response to AIDS and may have the only designated AIDS Program Office in corporate America. The in-house strategy is "top-down" beginning with senior managers who participate in a four-module program and then translate the flexible guidelines to employees. The AIDS Program Manager has continued to provide leadership to encourage other employers to adopt AIDS policies and programs, and the company continues to support the development of workplace educational materials (personal communication, P.A. Ross, Manager, *AIDS Program Office*, Digital Equipment Corp. 1991).

Syntex Corporation, an international pharamaceutical company based in California, began a proactive approach to AIDS in 1986, before any employee had been diagnosed with HIV/AIDS. Programs for managers/supervisors and employees include a video presenting the company's policies on employees with life-threatening illnesses and other issues. In promoting a proactive response among other companies, Syntex supported activities of the Business Leadership Task Force and participated in the video produced by the San Francisco AIDS Foundation to show how the AIDS program is implemented in their workplace. A senior executive contributed expertise in writing a brochure on the legal implications of AIDS in the workplace, published by the National Leadership Coalition on AIDS (Nau 1990).

J. P. Morgan and Company, a New York-based financial organization, began an AIDS education campaign in September 1987 conducted by the its medical department as part of its health promotion program. The voluntary sessions were attended by about one-tenth of the local employees, but "the feedback was very affirmative" (Schneider, Hair, and Jenkins 1989). Morgan has attempted to influence other organizations by surveying medical directors in similar large corporations about their AIDS policies and education efforts and by disseminating the results and the experience of their own program (Schneider et al. 1989; Schneider 1989).

Allstate Insurance Company (1988) provided visibility and focus for workplace AIDS concerns by sponsoring a 1987 conference, "AIDS: Corporate America Responds." More than 200 major companies met to learn more about the impact of AIDS on businesses and to take coordinated action. The detailed report serves as a guide to employers on legal and policy implications of AIDS in the workplace and gives resources for implementing policies and programs. A national survey of employers, sponsored jointly by *Fortune Magazine* (1988), has provided information on workplace activities and attitudes toward AIDS.

DISCUSSION

According to one analysis (Perrow and Guillen 1990), existing community and government organizations have failed in responding to HIV/AIDS (with a new organization developed in response to the epidemic a notable exception). This analysis could be applied to private-sector corporate organizations as well: bureaucratic or "normal" organizational failure; economic concerns; and ideology. First, employers are not positioned to act quickly in response to a health-care crisis; they have traditionally provided health benefits to enable employees to pay for health care and only recently have moved into the arena of health education, health promotion, and disease prevention (Barr 1991). Many employers have believed that AIDS is a disease affecting people not found in their own workforce, and they have not reacted until confronted directly by the problem.

Second, employers perceive that providing AIDS education is too costly and that raising the issues related to AIDS may "stir up" trouble and suggest, erroneously, that AIDS is a problem in the workplace; they have also worried about community image and prestige that could be "tarnished" if clients became concerned about AIDS in their workplace—another cost. Yet, companies such as IBM, Levi Strauss, and others have been identified with AIDS from the early days of the epidemic, making a public commitment. Economic motivation may encourage a workplace response when companies recognizing several HIV/AIDS cases consider the high costs of not addressing issues related to medical benefits and workplace disruption and the relative advantage of innovative responses to the "crisis" (Rogers 1983).

Third, ideology may have been a factor in that many of the early adopters were companies in San Francisco where efforts were linked to the work of the San Francisco AIDS Foundation, an organization that first responded to the needs and prevalence of AIDS in the gay community. Ideology also may be a factor in the denial expressed by employers. The earliest adopters were reactive; the ones starting after 1985 were more proactive. This sequence suggests that as awareness builds, employers may recognize that "it can happen here" and that it is in their own self-interest to clarify and communicate policies and to undertake education for managers and employees. Moreover, recent data indicate that a strong workplace education program is valued by employees as a more credible source of information about HIV/AIDS than the media and other sources (Barr and Warshaw 1990; Barr et al. 1991). Such findings may help convince employers that the costs of not acting may be much higher than the costs of a proactive response.

Government organizations have been slow to act. Yet, current efforts, especially at the federal level in the CDC, are mobilizing to encourage AIDS education in strategic locations throughout the nation (including areas just beginning to be affected by HIV/AIDS) and by small as well as large employers. Labor organizations are intensifying efforts to educate and protect employees, although they still lag in terms of widespread adoption. Providers of AIDS education for employers are recognizing that costs in time and resources are an issue for employers and that programs must be adapted to the needs of each worksite. At the same time, there appears to be greater acceptance of the expertise of specialized AIDS organizations and willingness to use them to provide education and training (Miller et al. 1990). Legislative imperatives may add to employers' readiness to adopt policies and programs; the Americans with Disabilities Act, in effect since July 1992, covers HIV/AIDS under its provisions for job accomodation and nondiscrimination inthe workplace.

That a number of private-sector AIDS coalitions have ceased to function suggests that the initial awareness stage of the innovation-decision process is slowing or possibly is complete enough to move into another phase. For example, the hierarchical model of diffusion of innovation being implemented by the National Leadership Coalition on AIDS begins with a leadership or "gatekeeper" organization, which endorses the innovation and passes it on to members; then, it is adopted by the rank and file membership in their own workplaces. This strategy uses existing lines of communication from the trade association to its members, many of which are minority and small businesses.

Recommendations for facilitating the diffusion of HIV/AIDS education to smaller organizations (Emery 1990) include: establish a focal point (i.e., a leadership organization), such as a Chamber of Commerce, to coordinate education activities; identify low-or/no-cost resources and materials that target workforces with different ethnic and other characteristics; work through local business networks to facilitate communication; and encourage the "mentoring" of large corporations to smaller businesses. One example of using existing networks is the video recently produced by the Los Altos (California) Rotary Club portraying its own experiences with members who themselves or whose family member has HIV/AIDS. This videotape is a strong motivator for employers to recognize that AIDS happens to people "like us" and that all must respond. It is being disseminated to Rotary clubs all over the world.[4]

Workplace HIV/AIDS policies and education programs represent not a technological innovation but a "social" innovation (Nathanson and Morlock 1980), with adoption linked to the values of the organization. While decentralization of power in organizations has been related to innovation (Kaluzny, Veney, and Gentry 1974; Aiken and Hage 1971), others have observed that social innovations occur more frequently where there is centralized decision making (Nathanson and Morlock 1980). Evidence to indicate that small companies where the CEO is the sole decision maker are less likely to have responded to AIDS in the workplace may be more a function of organizational size and resources than structure of decision making. The presence of a strong and committed internal leader has been an important factor in establishing AIDS policies and programs and may be critical in developing a proactive rather than reactive response (Miller et al. 1990).

The first phase of diffusion of AIDS policies and education was led by organizations composed of various companies linked by their interest and concern about AIDS and supported by existing agencies and key employers who were early adopters and acted as leaders to persuade others. As noted in the hierarchical model, a second phase of diffusion may focus on the specific environment of organizations in an institutional sector that could convey trust and legitimacy to AIDS activities (Meyer and Rowan 1977). While there is no clear "early majority" of employer organizations that have adopted HIV/ AIDS policies and programs, there may be a greater openness to such initiatives, providing the basis for their proliferation.

ACKNOWLEDGEMENTS

The thoughtful comments from Rosalind Brannigan and anonymous reviewers on an earlier version of this paper are gratefully acknowledged.

NOTES

1. This listing is not exhaustive of all types of organizations involved in some way in AIDS in the workplace. The purpose here is to present the major types of organizations that have played a leadership role to focus on some important examples.

2. Similarly, the American Management Association has distributed a handbook on AIDS to 25,000 human resources managers, and the National Association of Manufacturers, a founding member of the National Leadership Coalition on AIDS, has distributed a brochure for employees to its 13,000 members (Stiles 1988).

3. The American Red Cross is perhaps more widely known in relation to AIDS for its blood bank program and its commonly viewed early reluctance to deal with issues involved in testing the blood supply (Shilts 1987; Perrow and Guillen 1990).

4. Another singular leadership activity is that of Benneville Strohecker, a small business owner from Massachusetts, who took a year's sabbatical dedicated to promoting workplace AIDS policies and programs and served as consultant to the National Leadership Coalition on AIDS.

REFERENCES

Aiken, M. and J. Hage. 1971. "The Organic Organization and Innovation." *Sociology* 5: 63-82.
Allstate Insurance Company. 1988. *AIDS: Corporate America Responds.* Chicago: Allstate Insurance Company.
American Civil Liberties Union. 1990. *Epidemic of Fear.* New York: ACLU AIDS Project.
American Management Association. 1991. *1991 AMA Survey on Workplace Testing.* New York: American Management Association.
Ball, J.K., J.V. Kelly, and B.J. Turner. 1990. "Third-party Financing for AIDS Hospitalizations in New York." *AIDS Public Policy Journal* 5: 51-58.
Barr, J.K. 1991. "Employee Health Benefits: Corporate Strategies for Cost Containment." *Sociological Practice* 9: 120-140.
Barr, J.K. and L.J. Warshaw. 1990. *AIDS in the Workplace: What Employees Think.* New York: New York Business Group on Health.
Barr, J.K., J.M. Waring, and L.J. Warshaw. 1991. "Employees' Sources of AIDS Information: The Workplace as a Promising Educational Setting." *Journal of Occupational Medicine* 33: 143-147.
Bayer, R. 1989. *Private Acts, Social Consequences: AIDS and the Politics of Public Health.* New York: The Free Press.

Bayless, P. 1989. "AIDS at Work in NY: Fear, Evasion, Lawsuits." *Crain's New York Business* (March 20): 1.

Both, R.T. 1989. "When AIDS Calls Can You Respond?" *Corporate Report Wisconsin* (February): 13-15.

Business Roundtable. 1989. *A.I.D.S. Survey.* Washington, DC: Business Roundtable.

Citizen's Commission on AIDS for New York City and Northern New Jersey. 1987. *A Leadership Response to the Challenge of AIDS.* New York: Citizen's Commission on AIDS for New York City and Northern New Jersey.

_____. 1988. *Responding to AIDS: Ten Principles for the Workplace.* New York: Citizen's Commission on AIDS for New York City and Northern New Jersey.

Emery, A.R. 1990a. "Needs Assessment of Micro, Small, and Mid-sized Businesses and HIV/AIDS Education." Mimeo, San Francisco, July.

_____. 1990b. *The Next Step: HIV in the 90's–A Management Guide to AIDS in the Workplace.* San Francisco: San Francisco AIDS Foundation.

"Empire Blue Cross Ordered to Pay for Man's Bone Marrow Transplant" *AIDS Policy and Law* 5: 7.

Fielding, J.E. and P.V. Piserchia. 1989. "Frequency of Worksite Health Promotion Activities." *American Journal of Public Health* 79: 16-20.

Fortune Magazine and Allstate Insurance. 1988. *Business Response to AIDS: A National Survey of U.S. Companies.* New York: Time, Inc.

Foster Higgins. 1990. *Health Care Benefits Survey, 1989. Report 2: Indemnity Plans: Cost, Design and Funding.* Princeton, NJ: A. Foster Higgins and Co., Inc.

Gallagher, E.S. 1988. "Memo." San Francisco: Executive Leadership Council on AIDS, March 10.

Gurvitch, A.M. and S.M. Randolph. 1992. *HIV/AIDS Education in the Workplace: A National Survey of U.S. Small Businesses.* HIV/AIDS Monograph No.1. Washington, DC: American Red Cross.

Hardy, A.M. 1991. "AIDS Knowledge and Attitudes for October-December 1990: Provisional data from the National Health Interview Survey." Advance Data. No. 204. DHHS Pub. No. (PHS) 91-1250. Public Health Service. Hyattsville, MD: National Center for Health Statistics, July 1.

Haughie, G.E. 1987. "Confronting AIDS: Update on a Sensitive Issue." IBM Management Report, New York, September.

Hellinger, F.J. 1992. "Forecasts of the Costs of Medical Care for Persons with HIV: 1992-1995." *Inquiry* 29(Fall): 356-365.

Hollander, R.B. and J.J. Lengermann. 1988. "Corporate Characteristics and Worksite Health Promotion Programs: Survey Findings from Fortune 500 Companies." *Social Science and Medicine* 26: 491-501.

Holmes, S.L. 1977. "Corporate Social Performance: Past and Present Areas of Commitment." *Academy of Management Journal* 20: 433-438.

Kaluzny, A.D., J.E. Veney, and J.T. Gentry. 1974. "Innovation of Health Services: A Comparative Study of Hospitals." *Millbank Memorial Fund Quarterly/Health and Society* (Winter).

Kirp, D.L. 1989. "Uncommon Decency: Pacific Bell Responds to AIDS." *Harvard Business Review* (May-June): 140-151.

Landsbergis, P.A., R.L. Caplan, and M. Greenberg. 1991. "AIDS and Employment Policies: The Role of Labor Unions." *AIDS and Public Policy Journal* 6: 76-82.

Mattlin, J.A. 1988. *The Impact of AIDS on Philadelphia Businesses: Final Report on a Study of Area Businesses and Their Response to AIDS.* Reported prepared for the Philadelphia Commission on AIDS, Leonard Davis Institute of Health Economics, University of Pennsylvania. Philadelphia, PA: Institute for Survey Research, Temple University.

McHugh, W.F. 1989. *AIDS in the Workplace: Managing the AIDS Crisis.* Tallahassee, FL: Center for Employment Relations and Law, Florida State University.

Meyer J.W. and B. Rowan. 1983. "Institutionalized Organizations: Formal Structure as Myth and Ceremony." Pp. 21-44 in *Organizational Environments: Ritual and Rationality,* edited by J.W. Meyer and W.R. Scott. Beverly Hills, CA: Sage

Miller, R.L., J.K. Barr, S. Humes, L.J. Warshaw, and M. Reinfeld. 1990. "AIDS-Related Education and Training in the Workplace." New York: Gay Men's Health Crisis and The New York Business Group on Health, Inc.

Nathanson, C.A. and L.L. Morlock. 1980. "Control Structure, Values, and Innovation: A Comparative Study of Hospitals." *Journal of Health and Social Behavior* 21(December): 315-333

National AIDS Information Clearinghouse and National Leadership Coalition on AIDS. 1990. *AIDS and the Workplace: Resources for Workers, Managers, and Employers.* Atlanta, GA: Centers for Disease Control.

National Leadership Coalition on AIDS. 1990a. "CEOs Respond to AIDS." Mimeo. Washington, DC: National Leadership Coalition on AIDS.

————. 1990b. *Small Business and AIDS: How AIDS Can Affect Your Business.* Washington, DC: National Leadership Coalition on AIDS.

Nau, C. 1990. *The ADA and HIV: What Employers Need to Know Now.* Washington, DC: National Leadership Coalition on AIDS.

Netzer, B. 1991. "The 50 Best Clean and Green Investments." *MONEY* (June): 132-133.

New York Business Group on Health. 1989. "AIDS and the Workplace: A Legal/Regulatory Update." *Discussion Paper* 9, 1-12.

Ostlund, L.E. 1977. "Attitudes of Managers Toward Corporate Social Responsibility." *California Management Review* 19: 35-39.

Perrow, C. and M.F. Guillen. 1990. *The AIDS Disaster: The Failure of Organizations in New York and the Nation.* New Haven: Yale University Press.

Pickett, N.A., Jr., S.J. Drewry, and E.L. Comer. 1990. "AIDS: MetLife's Experience." *Statistical Bulletin* 71: 2-9.

Puckett, S.B. and A.R. Emery. 1988. *Managing AIDS in the Workplace.* Reading, MA: Addison-Wesley.

Rogers, E.M. 1983. *Diffusion of Innovations.* New York: The Free Press.

Schneider, W.J., M.R. Hait, and J.L. Jenkins. 1989. "The Corporate Medical Department and AIDS." *Bulletin of the New York Academy of Medicine* 65: 608-617.

Schneider, W.J. 1989. "AIDS in the Workplace." *Journal of Occupational Medicine* 31: 839-841.

Shilts, R. 1987. *And the Band Played On.* New York: Penguin Books.

Stiles, B.J. 1988. "How Should Businesses Respond to AIDS?" *AIDS Workplace Update* 1: 5-6.

UAW-GM Human Resource Center. 1988a. *Dealing with AIDS.* UAW-GM AIDS Information Network. Madison lHeights, MI: UAW-GM.

————. 1988b. AIDS Medical Videotape Library. Madison Heights, MI: UAW-GM.

Warshaw, L.J., ed. 1986. *AIDS and the Employer: Guidelines on the Management of AIDS in the Workplace.* New York: New York Business Group on Health, Inc.

Yellin, E.H., R.M. Greenblatt, H. Hollander, and J.R. McMaster. 1991. "The Impact of HIV-related Illness on Employment." *American Journal of Public Health* 81: 79-84.

STIGMA AND HOMECOMING:

FAMILY CAREGIVING AND THE "DISAFFILIATED" INTRAVENOUS DRUG USER

Stephen Crystal and Nina Glick Schiller

ABSTRACT

Persons with AIDS (PWAS) who have intravenous drug use histories, like IV drug users in general, have often been presumed to be socially disaffiliated. It is often assumed that they have exhausted conventional social resources such as those of family ties in the course of their drug-using career, leaving them with limited access to informal support in dealing with their illness. Data from a needs assessment study are used to illustrate the application of survey data to such questions; PWAs with IVDU histories appear to have no less access to family caregiving support than other PWAs. Conceptual and empirical issues in family caregiving in HIV illness are discussed; research on these topics represents a key issue on the agenda for social scientific AIDS research.

The Social and Behavioral Aspects of AIDS.
Advances in Medical Sociology, Volume 3, pages 165-184.
Copyright © 1993 by JAI Press Inc.
All Rights of reproduction in any form reserved.
ISBN: 1-55938-439-5

INTRODUCTION

Research on the care of persons with AIDS has focused predominantly on the provision of services through the formal health-care system. With AIDS increasingly taking on the attributes of a chronic illness, however, provision of nontechnical, supportive care to persons with AIDS (PWAs) has grown in importance. In other chronically ill or impaired populations, such as the functionally impaired elderly (Crystal 1984), research indicates that the majority of such care is provided through informal social networks (principally family) rather than through formal systems. Among the elderly, for example, the proportion with personal care dependency has been estimated at 15 to 20 percent, while only six percent receive care in nursing homes; of those residing in the community, formal services account for as little as 15 percent of the personal care provided (Doty, Liu, and Wiener 1985). Informal caregiving for the elderly is of great policy and fiscal importance since provision of comparable care through formal services would cost enormous sums.

A similar pattern of reliance on informal care provision exists in the case of AIDS, constituting an unheralded and uncompensated care delivery system of large scope and value, as well as a frequent source of severe strain for those called upon to provide the care. Indeed, formal care alternatives are often scarcer for PWAs than for other populations with chronic illness and functional impairment. In contrast to the major role played by nursing homes as a care source for the functionally impaired population, only a small proportion of PWAs receives care in nursing homes or other institutional long-term care facilities, for a variety of reasons including discrimination, reimbursement issues, and care preferences of PWAs themselves. Because of their predominantly geriatric orientation and population, existing facilities are typically unsuitable for a young adult population with an episodic rather than stable pattern of functional status; this creates additional pressure on informal care resources (Crystal 1989).

Some AIDS literature has emphasized the role, indeed an important one, of community volunteers (Arno 1986; Cline 1989; Scitovsky, Cline, and Lee 1986). However, this pattern of care, as epitomized by "buddy systems" and organizations such as San Francisco's Shanti Project or New York's Gay Men's Health Crisis, appears to be more widespread in large-city gay communities than elsewhere. With risk reduction proceeding more quickly in such communities than among more economically disadvantaged populations at risk, the profile of the epidemic is becoming geographically more dispersed and includes increasing proportions of persons with intravenous drug use (IVDU) histories, members of racial and ethnic minorities, and women. While community organization for self-help is possible among various at-risk groups including IVDUs (Friedman and Casriel 1988; Tenneriello et al. 1988; Watters 1989), the potential for large-scale implementation of volunteer-oriented peer support systems on the San Francisco model would appear to be more limited in economically stressed communities. For PWAs generally, and especially in such communities, families represent a central and often the most significant source of care provision. Such care provision extends both to instrumental and emotional support, and is provided both by conjugal families (spouses and partners) and by families of origin, most typically by parents.

While the issues involved in family caregiving to PWAs have much in common with those studied in previous work on caregiving—most of which has focused on the elderly—there are important differences as well (Crystal 1989; Benjamin 1988). Among the most important of these is the reversal of generational perspective. While family caregiving of the elderly usually involves the older generation being cared for by the younger, the reverse is often true in connection with AIDS (O'Donnell et al. 1990). Although there are many young adults with chronic illness, much less systematic research has been done on family caregiving for this diverse population. The affliction of a substantial population of young adults with chronic illness caused by HIV raises a new set of problems for family caregiving. Parents and other older family members face the crisis of an ill adult child, presenting caregiving demands that compete with other responsibilities (Allers 1990). Issues presented include the rearrangement of households and renegotiation of relationships often strained by conflicting lifestyle choices and values.

The pervasive presence of stigma associated with HIV illness and the need to manage stigma constitute another distinctive factor in AIDS caregiving. Most persons with AIDS, whether IVDU, homosexual, or members of other "risk groups," are subject to pervasive stigma adhering to their risk-group membership and to the disease itself; multiple discrediting characteristics are attributed to them. In his well-known analysis of the social process of stigmatization, Goffman (1963) classifies such sources of social discredit into three types, all of which apply to the PWA's situation: abominations of the body (as with the purple marks of Kaposi's Sarcoma), blemishes of character (such as weak will or unnatural passions), and tribal stigmata of a despised group. Conrad (1986) has observed, "It would be difficult to imagine a scenario for a more stigmatizing disease," combining the elements of contagiousness, sexual transmissibility, and deadly outcome. Prevalent images of AIDS evoke deeply rooted fears and anxieties connected with death and sexuality (Sontag 1989), which may be expressed in the form of exaggerated fear of contagion through casual contact. Distancing or rejection by some of the members of one's social network is a common experience for PWAs (Crystal and Jackson 1989). Within already-stigmatized groups such as communities of gay men, the crisis of the illness has, for some, increased group solidarity expressed through volunteerism, activism and other collective responses. Others, however, distance themselves from infected peers. One ethnographic study of gay men, for example, describes the ways in which the uninfected limit or avoid contact with PWAs through physical and emotional distancing, as well as through the adoption of self-concepts which construct social boundaries from the infected (Kowalewski 1988).

AIDS' association with behavior perceived as morally dangerous adds to its stigma; Poirier (1988) describes the stigmatization of persons with AIDS as resulting from the fear not of physical but of moral contagion, and Herek and Glunt (1988) refer to it as an "epidemic of stigma." This process can take on much the same quality as, in societies with caste systems, the attribution of ritual impurity to the low-caste from whom one must keep one's distance. Such symbolic stigma can spread to families and other close associates—a process described by Goffman as courtesy stigma. While some family members become involved in caregiving, PWAs experience rejection by others (Crystal and Jackson 1989); in some instances, instrumental caregiving can coexist with disapproval, emotional or physical distancing, or anger over past behavior. For PWAs with an IV drug use history, disappointment and family strains related to past or perhaps continuing drug use can be an important issue affecting family caregiving.

INTRAVENOUS DRUG USERS WITH AIDS—SOCIAL DISAFFILIATES?

While research on informal caregiving among urban gay white PWAs has been limited, even less is known with respect to other PWA populations. Individuals with intravenous drug use histories (IVDUs), for example, account for an increasingly large proportion of cases. IVDUs are commonly viewed as socially disaffiliated and isolated from conventional social structures and sources of social support, as a result of their problematic and illegal lifestyles. It is assumed that they have often exhausted social resources in the course of their drug-using career, leaving them with limited access to informal support in dealing with their illness (Macklin 1988). They are viewed by some researchers as very difficult subjects for social and health research because of unstable lifestyles and residential patterns (Glenn 1989; Smith 1989).

IVDUs' interpersonal relationships are presumed to be strained by prevalent pathologies of personality such as antisocial personality disorder— characterized as, among other features, being unable to form meaningful relationships and as having superficial and very unstable interpersonal relationships (Gerstley, Alterman, McLellan, and Woody 1990; Youngstrom 1991). It has been asserted, for example, that about 40 percent of patients entering methadone maintenance, and a similar proportion of IVDUs not in drug treatment, can be classified as having antisocial personality disorder (Gerstley, Alterman, McLellan, and Woody 1990; Rounsaville and Kleber 1985); in one study of treated addicts the proportion was 54 percent

(Rounsaville, Weissman, Kleber, and Wilber 1982). It is suggested that the proportion is even higher among IVDUs with AIDS, since sociopathic personality structure is argued to be associated with higher rates of high-risk behavior such as needlesharing (Brooner et al. 1990). In one study, 64 percent of IVDUs with HIV infection were categorized as having "antisocial personality disorder" (Youngstrom 1991). In this view, the epidemiological processes associated with HIV transmission would be seen as a filter selecting the most socially marginal, deviant drug users.

Based on these views of IVDUs with AIDS, we might expect to find little involvement in conventional roles and social structures on their part. Since images of street drug culture have been associated particularly with drug use in the black community, this might be expected to be even more the case in areas in which many IVDUs are black. Research on the actual social context of IVDUs' lives has been scarce and has focused mostly on the drug-using behavior itself and its immediate setting and antecedents. A long-standing tradition in sociological work on drug addiction, stemming in part from the influential work of Lindesmith (1968), interpreted substance use by addicts as a sociopsychological phenomenon sharply distinct from substance use by nonaddicts. Opiate addicts were viewed as quickly entering into, in their drug-using career, an addicted state in which drugs were used not for pleasure-seeking but to avoid withdrawal symptoms. This tradition facilitated the image of the addict as "not like you or me." Evidence that severe physical habituation did not always coexist with chronic drug use and that opiate use often represented not just symptom alleviation, but a pleasure-seeking behavior not so different from other forms of substance use (McAuliffe and Gordon 1975), was often resisted or denied. Along similar lines, the existence of a population of recurrent casual users, less physically addicted than psychologically habituated, was also downplayed in favor of the dope fiend stereotype.

In addition to biased perspectives deriving from reliance on theoretical constructs which emphasized physiological addiction, data-availability biases contributed to the perception of addicts as being far removed from the social mainstream. The most visible and accessible addicts have been those who came into contact with the criminal justice system; those who hit bottom and entered treatment; and conspicuous street addicts. Those who managed to maintain aspects of conventional social existence, such as legitimate employment, constituted a harder-to-study population.

The wave of ethnographic research on drug use that has emerged since the start of the AIDS epidemic, prompted by concern about prevention of transmission through needle-sharing, has not substantially changed this picture since this work too has largely focused on social behavior surrounding the drug use itself, emphasizing "street life" (DesJarlais and Friedman 1987). Thus, this work has also tended to perpetuate the perception of IVDUs as living lives which are separate and apart from nondrug-using society. Studies focusing attention on street life and the street addict role have emphasized the powerful influence of a street subculture of heroin users, which provides a blueprint for living for many users (Stephens 1991) and serves as a social identity around which behavior is pervasively organized. While providing a more sociologically sophisticated perspective on drug users' behavior than offered by theories that reduce the complex social behavior surrounding drug use to personality pathology or pharmacology, work in this genre still perpetuates an incomplete image of users' social worlds by narrowing the focus to street life and to the social behavior immediately involved in drug use.

Social-scientific views of IVDUs which emphasize their "differentness" are in many respects parallel to images held by health care personnel and others involved in AIDS care delivery (Gee 1989). Persons with IVDU histories are widely seen as difficult to care for, noncompliant with treatment regimens and clinic attendance, lacking social supports, manipulative, and not truly interested in recovery from addiction. PWAs with such backgrounds have often been viewed as less appropriate for community-based care programs than other PWAs. Indeed, while negative attitudes toward both homosexuals as well as IVDUs have been found to be widely held among health professionals (Schwartz 1989), it appears reasonable to conclude that with respect to IVDUs such views are more strongly held, felt to be more socially acceptable, and more likely to affect care. There has been less focus on their needs. It is therefore not surprising that IVDUs with AIDS have been found less likely to be offered treatment such as Zidovudine (AZT) which is expensive and requires close medical monitoring and patient compliance (Stein et al. 1991).

DIMENSIONS OF AIDS CAREGIVING

Clearly, stigmatization creates an additional barrier for family caregiving for PWAs. The economic pressures faced by most PWAs, and many of their families, create another set of barriers. Their income typically drops precipitously (Crystal and Jackson 1989; Carwein and Ray 1989); if they are members of racial or ethnic communities under economic pressure, few family financial resources may be available.

Under these pressures, many apparent barriers confront family caregiving, and it might well be presumed to be an endangered species of behavior. At the same time, the analogy with other chronically ill populations suggests the important role family care can play. Economic disadvantage, for example, need not function as a deterrent; families often rise to the occasion of financial need. Among economically stressed black Americans, numerous studies have documented the presence of strong extended family help structures, with exchange of services in coresidential households which help family members cope with limited financial resources (Martin and Martin 1978; Stack 1974).

As with the elderly, coresident family constitute an important though certainly not the only source of informal instrumental assistance. Thus, living arrangements are one key indicator of potential care resources. In most cases, the presence of coresident family members does imply access to some degree of instrumental assistance with such matters as shopping, meal preparation, and household maintenance, and often with personal care if needed as well. It is important, however, to note that the presence of coresident family members does not *assure* the provision of needed instrumental services (let alone emotional support), and should be considered an indicator of *potential* access to care.

The care needs of persons with AIDS include many varieties of instrumental assistance, such as help with household maintenance; perhaps as important are the emotional needs, not only for reassurance but for support in coming to terms with having a fatal illness, in maintaining self-esteem, and in maintaining a sense of control over one's life (Adelman 1989). The distinction between instrumental and emotional support is important in studying AIDS caregiving since one does not necessarily coincide with the other. Instrumental support may be provided out of a sense of necessity without always being accompanied by a positive emotional relationship between the caregiver and care recipient. Resentment over caretaking burdens, past or present substance use, or behavior seen as leading to the infection can affect the quality of the relationship. Emotional closeness, where it exists, may not be uniformly positive in nature; codependency, for example, is a risk of such caregiving situations.

The role of the family in AIDS caregiving is of obvious policy importance. It has, however, been the focus of surprisingly little research. This is in part because epidemiological and biomedical concerns have so strongly outweighed those surrounding AIDS care in the setting of research agendas. It also has to do with the difficulty experienced by researchers in generating representative samples of persons with AIDS for social research and the cost of implementing such research. For these and other reasons, systematic knowledge has been scarce in this area.

Research needs to begin with basic descriptive information on the extent of family caregiving for persons with AIDS and the family forms in which it is provided. What, for example, are the roles of families of origin (consanguineal families) as compared with those of conjugal families? To what extent is help provided through coresidential arrangements, and to what extent by family members outside the coresidential household? Answers to these and other questions have been slow to emerge.

The need for better understanding of informal caregiving in the HIV epidemic suggests the importance of well-designed empirical research in this area. The research agenda suggested by these needs is diverse and encompasses both instrumental and emotional dimensions of support. To understand variations in informal caregiving, it is also necessary to place them in the context of variations in help needs and receipt of formal services. Of particular importance is empirical research on family caregiving which makes possible comparison across the major subgroups within the PWA population nationally. While gay white men represented a high proportion of cases early in the epidemic and were often the principal focus of attention, other subgroups now represent a growing share of the affected population. In particular, intravenous drug use accounts for an increasing proportion of cases. Do PWAs with IVDU histories seem distinctively "disaffiliated" and lacking in social supports?

An example of the sort of empirical data which can illustrate family caregiving patterns is provided by data from a 1989-90 survey of persons with AIDS in New Jersey. The data presented in the Tables and discussed below focus primarily on the instrumental dimension of support. The focus here is on indicators of informal, instrumental support for IVDUs and, for comparison, those of other subgroups.

METHODS

The study was funded by and undertaken with the cooperation of the New Jersey Department of Health, in large part for needs-assessment purposes. At the state's request, we undertook to investigate the feasibility of developing a statewide sample of persons with AIDS, using as a sample frame the state AIDS registry, maintained for surveillance purposes by the Department of Health. The State was particularly interested in a registry-based sample so that patients served by the whole spectrum of health care providers, and those unconnected or only loosely connected to the care system, could be included.

To carry out this study, we developed a protocol under which participation was invited by the health provider if possible, by the surveillance office if that was not possible, or when necessary by the research team. The protocol and procedures were reviewed by Institutional Review Boards for the Department, for Rutgers University, and for one of the major cooperating hospitals in the state. Because of the sensitive nature of information about HIV illness, a Certificate of Confidentiality was applied for and received from the United States Public Health Service.

This approach was expected to, and did, require a protracted and difficult effort in order to recruit a study population. However, it provided a statewide sample of respondents served by a range of health providers, as well as those not utilizing health care during a particular period. It provided us with the ability to assess whether biases from differential response rates were present, since characteristics of noninterviewed as well as interviewed sample members were known.

Table 1. Demographic Profile
(In Percent)

	Total New Jersey[a] (n = 2,759)	Random Sample (n = 475)	Interviewed Respondents (n = 107)
Gender			
Male	77	77	75
Female	23	23	25
Race/Ethnicity			
White	34	34	36
Black	53	52	49
Hispanic	13	14	15
Asian	*	1	1
Mode of Transmission			
Homosexual/bisexual	27	25	28
Intravenous drug use	56	56	55
Homosexual/intravenous	3	4	6
Heterosexual	9	12	8
Transfusion/hemophilia	2	3	4
Other	3	1	—
Age			
20-29 years	19	21	18
30-39 years	52	53	48
40-49 years	19	20	25
50+ years	6	6	9

Notes: [a] Profile of individuals in New Jersey Registry not known to have died as of October 1989.
        * Less than 1 percent

A sample of persons who had been reported with full-blown AIDS (as defined by the Centers for Disease Control) and who were not known to have subsequently died was drawn in four waves between October 1988 and October 1989, totaling 475 cases (see Table 1). Of these, 115 or 24 percent were determined by subsequent investigation to have fallen outside the sampling criteria because they had died before the date on which their names were drawn. Of the 360 remaining cases in the sample, 45 were determined to have moved out of state or to have had their records closed to further contact at the request of the reporting provider, leaving 315. We successfully located and interviewed 107 of these 315 cases; the major loss was inability to locate, while most of those contacted agreed to be interviewed.

A particularly significant aspect of this study is that it represents the population of PWAs in a state where the proportion of intravenous drug users (IVDUs), of minorities, and of women is high compared to national data and to many of the sites for previous AIDS health services research. Since these subgroups are all increasing as a proportion of persons with AIDS in the United States, the sample provides insight into the present and indeed the future of the epidemic which is not available from populations where gay white men predominate. Table 1 indicates the demographic characteristics of not-known-dead persons with AIDS as of October 1989 in New Jersey (from Registry data), as well as the demographic characteristics of the sample of names drawn from the Registry and the respondents we interviewed. The interviewed sample was quite similar demographically to the original sample and to the total population of persons reported to the Registry, with no significant differences on demographic variables. The proportion of black or Hispanic people in the final interviewed sample was 64 percent as compared with 66 percent in Registry data. The proportion of IV drug users was 61 percent as compared with 59 percent in Registry data.

Detailed social histories were obtained during a comprehensive interview which took about three hours and was in many instances completed in two installments. The study was designed primarily to evaluate needs by assessing such information as functional status, economic and housing circumstances, access to informal care, and benefit utilization. Social support data were collected by self-report.

FINDINGS

Of the 107 respondents, 65 or 61 percent had intravenous drug use histories: of these, six were gay male IVDUs and the remaining 59 were categorized as IVDU only. Analyses were conducted with the gay IVDUs grouped with the other IVDUs and with the other gay men, with generally similar results; in the tables in the present paper, they are grouped with the other IVDUs. There were 30 non-IVDU gay men and 12 cases in other risk groups, which included both transfusion-related cases and those assumed to be heterosexually acquired. Seventy-five percent were men and 25 percent women. Forty-nine percent were black, 15 percent Hispanic, and 36 percent non-Hispanic white. Sixty-three percent of whites and the same proportion of blacks had IVDU histories. Forty-two percent of respondents had less than a high school education while 13 percent were college graduates; thus, this group was less elducationally advantaged than the poulations studied in much of the previous social and health services research on persons with AIDS. They presented 18 of the State's 21 counties, with the best-presented being Essex County, which includes Newark, and Hudson County, which includes Jersey City. It is also worth noting that this was not a geographically mobile population. Only four percent had lived in New Jersey less than five years and only 13 percent 10 years or less; most had lived in the state their whole life.

Table 2. Living Arrangements by Ethnicity, Risk Group, and Gender

	Alone or with Minor Children Only		Consanguineous Family		Family of Commitment (Spouse/ Life Partner)		Other		Total	
	n	%	n	%	n	%	n	%	n	%
Total	22	20.8	43	40.6	25	23.6	16	15.1	106	100
Ethnicity										
White, non-Hispanic	6	15.8	16	42.1	12	31.6	4	10.5	38	100
Black	12	23.1	23	44.2	8	15.4	9	17.3	52	100
Hispanic	4	25.0	4	25.0	5	31.3	3	18.8	16	100
Black/Hispanic	16	23.5	27	39.7	13	19.1	12	17.6	68	100
Risk Group*										
IVDU	7	10.8	32	49.2	15	23.1	11	16.9	65	100
Homosexual male	10	33.3	8	26.7	7	23.3	5	16.7	30	100
Other (hetero/transf)	5	41.7	3	25.0	3	25.0	1	8.3	12	100
Total non-IVDU	5	35.7	11	26.2	10	23.8	6	14.3	42	100
Gender										
Male	15	18.8	29	36.3	22	27.5	14	17.5	80	100
Female	7	25.9	14	51.9	3	11.1	3	11.1	27	100

Notes: * For IVDU versus non-IVDU, $p(x^2) = .011$
For IVDU versus homosexual male, $p(x^2) = .039$

Among the IVDUs, who are a particular focus of the present analysis, fewer than half had completed high school. Forty-eight percent were in their thirties and 37 percent were over 40, with 15 percent under 30. Sixty-four percent received Medicaid and 16 percent had private insurance, but 21 percent had no health care coverage. Median income was under $6,000, so this was a group with particularly substantial economic and educational disadvantage. A major indicator of potential informal help availability is provided by data on living arrangements. Notwithstanding the isolated or disaffiliated image, IVDUs were significantly less likely than others to be living alone. Table 2 shows that only 11 percent of IVDUs, versus 33 percent of gay men, were living alone. About half, 49 percent, of IVDUs were living with parents or other family of origin, as compared with 27 percent of gay men. Twenty-three percent of gay men and the same percentage of IVDUs were living with a spouse or life partner. (There were only three cases in which the PWA was living both with family of origin and a life partner; these cases were classified according to the principal informal-care provider, who was the life partner or spouse in each case). Consanguineous family was the most common living arrangement both for men and for women with AIDS, and both for blacks and for whites.

Table 3.　Social Support by Risk Group

	IVDU		Homosexual Men		Other		Total Non-IVDU		Total	
	n	%	n	%	n	%	n	%	n	%
Contact with kin in last week										
Yes	45	69.2	23	76.7	9	75.0	32	76.2	77	72.0
Base	65		30		12		42		107	
Has someone to get reassurance from										
Yes	47	74.6	22	78.6	9	75.0	31	77.5	78	75.7
Base	63		28		12		40		103	
Has someone to talk to about thoughts/feelings										
Yes	37	60.7	21	75.0	5	41.7	26	65.0	63	62.4
Base	61		28		12		40		101	
Has someone to talk to About problems										
Yes	45	71.4	22	75.9	6	50.0	28	68.3	73	70.2
Base	63		29		12		41		104	

Table 3 provides data on other aspects of social support by risk group. Similar proportions of both groups had had contact with kin in the last week, reported having someone to get reassurance from, said they had someone to talk to about thoughts and feelings, and reported having someone to talk to about their problems. None of the small differences on these indicators were statistically significant. Table 4 provides information on a more concrete dimension of assistance, help with the activities of daily living (such as bathing and dressing) and with "instrumental activities of daily living" (such as shopping for food, keeping the house clean, and preparing meals). Twenty percent of IVDUs and the same proportion of gay men had one or more unmet ADL needs; the proportions with at least one unmet IADL need, at 15 percent for IVDUs and 13 percent for gay men, were also similar. IVDUs were also no less likely than gay men to perceive that caregiving support would be available in the future when needed.

Respondents were asked if there was one main person who provided help and, if so, who that person was (Table 5). For IVDUs, the sources of help were predominantly family members and particularly family of origin. Among IVDU respondents reporting a single primary helper, spouses and life partners accounted for 24 percent while mothers accounted for 31 percent and other family for 38 percent. Among gay men, life partners accounted for 33 percent

Table 4. Unmet ADL and IADL Needs by Risk Group

	IVDU		Homosexual Men		Other		Total Non-IVDU		Total	
	n	%	n	%	n	%	n	%	n	%
Unmet ADL Needs										
Yes	13	20.0	6	20.0	5	41.7	11	26.2	24	22.4
Base	65		30		12		42		107	
Unmet IADL Needs										
Yes	10	15.4	4	13.3	4	33.3	8	19.0	18	16.8
Base	65		30		12		42		107	

and mothers another 33 percent; there were no "other family," while friends accounted for 27 percent. Only one IVDU and one gay man reported that the main person who helped was a professional care provider. Thus, while IVDUs and gay men were about equally likely to report that a spouse was their main helper, other family members were more likely to be the main helper for IVDUs; these were mainly family-of-origin kin.

DISCUSSION

A substantial body of gerontological research has documented the crucial role of families in the care of those elderly with chronic illness or impairment. Results of the present study indicate that this is also true for persons with AIDS: informal caregiving, largely through family, plays a vital part in their care and extends across risk group, race, and gender. Despite the stigma associated both with the illness and with the risk-group statuses which account for the majority of PWAs, families (particularly families of origin) provide a substantial level of social and instrumental support for a large proportion of PWAs. This does not mean, of course, that a stronger system of formal care is not urgently needed to complement families in these roles and to provide care when families are nonexistent or unavailable. It is important, however, that public policies take account of existing family support systems and function in cooperation with them rather than at cross purposes to them.

Particularly important, and scarce in much of the previous research, are the data on family support systems of IVDUs with AIDS. Sociological views of IV drug users have often characterized them as socially disaffiliated and as lacking social ties to the nondrug-using world. As discussed in the introductory section, they are frequently seen as having exhausted social resources and as having superficial and very unstable interpersonal relationships. Some

Table 5.   Relationship to Primary Helper (Among Respondents
Reporting a Single Primary Helper)

Relationship to Primary Helper	IVDU		Homosexual Men		Other		Total Non-IVDU		Total	
	n	%	n	%	n	%	n	%	n	%
Mother	13	31.0	5	33.3	2	25.0	7	30.4	20	30.8
Other Family	16	38.1	0	0.0	3	37.5	3	13.0	19	29.2
Life Partner/Spouse	10	23.8	5	33.3	1	12.5	6	26.1	16	24.6
Friend	2	4.8	4	26.7	1	12.5	5	21.7	7	10.8
Professional	1	2.4	1	6.7	1	12.5	2	8.7	3	4.6
Total	42	100.0	15	100.0	8	100.0	23	100.0	65	100.0

researchers have labeled IVDUs as commonly characterized by antisocial personality disorder and its accompanying pathologies of interpersonal relationships, and argued that this is even more prevalent among those who acquire HIV, since IVDUs with the riskiest drug-use behavior, such as frequent needle-sharing, are the most likely to become infected.

Certainly, many IVDUs may have brought much grief to their families through their drug use. For those who become ill with AIDS, however, this does not mean that their families are not there for them. As our data indicate, they appear to have access to family support which is comparable to that received by other PWAs. Parents and other family-of-origin members are the principal source of this help. IVDUs were no more likely than other PWAs to have unmet personal care needs, and were actually significantly less likely to be living alone and more likely to be living in family settings.

The family support received by PWAs in our study, extending across risk groups, highlights the enduring functionality of family support systems in responding to the needs of family members even under conditions of great strain. IVDUs with AIDS are exposed to very high levels of stigma associated with multiple discredited statuses. They experience substantial episodic impairments and the burden of multiple chronic symptoms such as fatigue, weakness, diarrhea, and night sweats, with fluctuating levels of needs that are likely to create substantial burdens on coresident family members and informal caregivers. Caregiving families taking kin with AIDS into their homes might also face secondary stigma from friends and neighbors. With median income less than $6,000, and with only 8 percent having income of as much as $10,000, subjects were impoverished, thus being likely to be an economic as well as a care burden to family. Family relationships had often been strained over the years by the subject's drug use. Nevertheless, and in the face of these barriers, substantial social and instrumental support had materialized in most cases from family members, particularly from consanguineal kin, most often a mother or other female kin. In contrast, friends, buddies, and community volunteers appeared to play a more limited role. Even among the gay men, most support came from family of origin and from life partners (whom we classed as conjugal family), rather than from friends or buddies.

As with the functionally impaired elderly population, the presence of an active, informal family support system should not be taken to argue against the need for comprehensive formal support systems. These systems are properly seen as complementary rather than competing, and significant gaps still remain, as witness the 20 percent reporting one or more unmet needs with activities of daily living. It should also be noted that, as with the elderly, instrumental support and emotional support do not necessarily go hand in hand. In some of the families, provision of physical care seemed to be associated with a significant degree of emotional strain or even open anger. Strain might be particularly severe if drug use was continuing, as acknowledged by 27 percent of our IVDU respondents, a figure which should be considered as a minimum proportion.

Notwithstanding these caveats, however, the extensive role played by family caregiving, extending across risk groups, is clearly indicated in the findings from this patient survey. The data presented in the tables on indicators of instrumental assistance suggest that both popular and social-scientific stereotypes about social disaffiliation of intravenous drug users can mislead. Similar divergence from stereotypes has been noted in other research: for example, a New York study of IVDUs by DesJarlais and colleagues found that 23 percent of respondents were employed, including some upper middle-class professionals (Goldsmith 1991). In addition to misperception of informal caregiving resources, such stereotypes might foster underestimation of IVDUs' ability to modify risky behavior in response to educational intervention or programs to provide clean needles, and could engender an unduly negative view of their ability to follow through on treatment regimens.

Stereotypical views of members of HIV "risk groups" are, of course, pervasive, not only with respect to IVDUs but with respect to gay men and others as well. In fact, these groups are highly diverse; survey research like the present study highlights the heterogeneity within these subpopulations of PWAs as well as within subpopulations defined in terms of race or ethnicity. Publicity associated with the AIDS epidemic has influenced perceptions of social behavior among gay men in complex and diverse ways. On the one hand, the impressive community self-help efforts in big-city gay communities like New York and San Francisco have dramatized the superficiality of stereotypes of gay men as more interested in individualistic pleasure-seeking than in social responsibility. On the other hand, publicity from early epidemiological studies and controversies over issues such as bathhouses promoted stereotypes of promiscuous lifestyles. In the politics of AIDS, such stereotyping has in common with the stereotyping of IVDUs the function of creating social distance from members of these risk groups, from the threat of the epidemic itself, and from the fears and responsibilities associated with it. The locution commonly employed in discussion of the possible expansion of transmission through heterosexual contact—"spread to the general population" (as though gay men and IVDUs were not part of the general population)—illustrates distancing of this kind. The distancing impulse has sometimes led to denial of the very possibility of extensive heterosexual spread (Fumento 1990).

Understandably, much social research on HIV illness has focused on the behaviors most directly related to virus transmission: sexual contact and IV drug use. As noted above, for example, even recent anthropological accounts of IV drug users which aim to place their social behavior into context often have focused on "street life," the mechanics of drug acquisition and use, shooting galleries, and social relationships with fellow users—a focus which has helped perpetuate stereotypes of disaffiliation from more conventional social ties. Surveys of IVDUs in the literature often have a similar emphasis (Friedman et al. 1985). Similarly, in epidemiological research on HIV among gay men, the concentration of attention on the specifics of sexual acts—often reminiscent of the early Kinsey studies—has sometimes decontextualized these social behaviors and contributed to stereotyping. What has usually been missing has been research which places persons with or at risk of HIV illness in a broader social context of family, community, and other ties, in common with "the rest of us."

The data presented here, while illustrative of some of the kinds of questions that can be addressed by survey data on persons with HIV illness, focus mainly on instrumental support and on a limited set of indicators. Much more work is needed to characterize the multiple dimensions of social support in HIV illness by family, as broadly defined. Patterns of variation in family structure, and the associated variations in function, need to be explored in greater depth. In this discussion, for example, for the purpose of broad description, domestic partnerships of gay men have been grouped with heterosexual marital and nonmarital domestic partnerships in the conjugal kin category. Much more needs to be understood, however, about the variations in structure and function of such ties. In the particular context of HIV illness, it is important to understand (across risk groups) the impact of illness on conjugal ties and the circumstances under which such ties do or do not endure through the course of the illness. The relationship between living arrangements and support (instrumental and emotional) needs to be better understood, and such understanding is best provided in relation to the course of the disease. For example, living alone may or may not represent absence of social support; shared living arrangements may tend to be initiated later in the course of illness when instrumental help needs increase, or such individuals may have access to support from non-coresident persons.

A complex set of questions revolves around the family's role in providing emotional support and the effect of such support on a variety of outcomes, including morbidity and mortality. As noted, instrumental and emotional support need not coexist; willingness to meet urgent instrumental needs does not necessarily mean that relationships are not strained and conflictual. Not infrequently, work on social support has conceptualized it as a unidimensional phenomenon which could be operationalized through portmanteau scales that mix many different sorts of interactions. Much work needs to be done to differentiate the dimensions of social support among PWAs and their interrelationships, and to investigate the applicability of schemata developed in work on other populations.

One paradigm which has frequently been articulated at the theoretical level, but which has been difficult to test rigorously, focuses on the effect of social support as a buffer for the effects of stress on the immune system, with a resulting positive impact on survival and morbidity (Kaplan, Johnson, Bailey, and Simon 1987). Such effects are likely to be difficult to detect because of the complex and multidimensional nature of social support and because of the many other sources of variation in morbidity and mortality which would need to be controlled for. An alternative route by which family and other sources of social support affect illness outcomes involves their role as intermediaries in access to and utilization of medical care and other formal services. With the development of treatment regimens which appear to have significant impact on survival, but which produce side effects and require careful medical management, it is likely that patients with support in negotiating the care system may differ from others in terms of access to and utilization of care, with possible effects on "hard" biological outcomes. This role requires much more extensive investigation. More generally, the relationship between formal and informal service provision in HIV illness has been little explored.

Whether or not family and other social support influences survival, it certainly seems reasonable to expect that it affects psychological coping with the impact of illness, and thus psychological well-being and quality of life. Clearly, PWAs must deal with a variety of stressors including the physical impact of illness, knowledge of limited life expectancy, rejection and discrimination, economic disadvantage, and others. In the face of these stresses, many become severely depressed. Significantly, however, many do manage to maintain a relatively positive mood and mobilize positive coping strategies. The role of family support in this process is a key research question.

Finally, research needs to focus not only on the impact of care provision on persons with HIV illness but also on the impact on those providing care. Caregiver-burden studies have attracted a great deal of interest in gerontological research over the last decade. Little is known, however, about the impact of caregiving on families in the HIV context, where parents,

182   STEPHEN CRYSTAL and NINA GLICK SCHILLER

grandparents, siblings, and other family of origin kin take on stressful caregiving responsibilities for an ill young adult.

In gerontological research, work of the 1960s and 1970s often challenged the myth of the isolated nuclear family with findings showing the continued strength of extended family structures in provision of social support and caregiving. An occupational risk for social scientists is to exaggerate counterstereotype findings into new, overly simplified, countervailing perspectives, as sometimes happened in gerontology with the rediscovery of the "unimpaired extended family." It is important that findings on the strength of informal support systems not be misconstrued to deemphasize real and unmet needs, particularly in a population disadvantaged by lack of adequate access to income support, health care coverage, and a host of other necessary resources (Crystal and Jackson 1989). On the other hand, formal services need to take account of existing informal support systems, particularly parents and other family-of-origin kin who appear to play the most substantial role in informal caregiving. Rather than either ignoring or taking for granted informal caregivers, service models can be designed to complement and support them. As in other chronically ill populations, families constitute a resource of crucial importance in dealing with the needs and limitations imposed by illness. Variations in informal caregiving, and their relationship to formal systems of care provision, constitute a topic of vital importance for social research on HIV illness, with important implications for program design.

REFERENCES

Adelman, M. 1989. "Social Support and *AIDS." AIDS and Public Policy Journal* 4(1): 31-9.
Allers, C.T. 1990. "AIDS and the Older Adult." *The Gerontologist* 30(3): 405-407.
Arno, P. 1986. "The Nonprofit Sector's Response to the AIDS Epidemic: Community-based Services in San Francisco." *American Journal of Public Health* 76(11): 1325-1330.
Benjamin, A.E. 1988. "Long-term Care and AIDS: Perspectives from Experience with the Elderly." *Milbank Quarterly* 66(3): 415-443.
Brooner, R.K, et al. 1990. "Intravenous Drug Abusers with Antisocial Personality Disorder: Increased HIV Risk Behavior." *Drug Alcohol Depend* 26(1)(Aug): 39-44.
Carwein, V.L. and C.G. Ray. 1989. "AIDS-related Income Losses and Implications for Policy Making." *Aids and Public Policy Journal* 4(2): 106-111.
Cline, R. 1989. "Communication and Death and Dying: Implications for Coping with AIDS." *AIDS and Public Policy Journal* 4(1): 40-50.
Conrad, P. 1986. "The Social Meaning of AIDS." *Social Policy* (Summer): 51-56.
Crystal, S. 1984. *America's Old Age Crisis: Public Policy and the Two Worlds of Aging.* Rev. ed. New York: Basic Books.
————, 1989. "Persons with AIDS and Older People: Common Long-term Care Concerns." Pp. 147-166 in *AIDS in an Aging Society: What We Need to Know,* edited by M.W. Riley, M. Ory, and D. Zablotsky. New York: Springer.
Crystal, S. and M. Jackson. 1989. "Psychosocial Adaptation and Economic Circumstances of Persons with AIDS and AIDS-related Complex." *Family and Community Health* 12(2): 77-88.

DesJarlais, D. and S. Friedman. 1987. "HIV Infection Among Intravenous Drug Users: Epidemiology and Risk Reduction." *AIDS* 1.

Doty, P. K. Liu, and J. Wiener. 1985. "An Overview of Long-term Care." *Health Care Financing Review* 6: 69-78.

Friedland, G.H., C. Harris, C. Butkus-Small, D. Shine, B. Moll, W. Darrow, and R.S. Klein. 1985. *Archives of Internal Medicine* 145: 1413-1417.

Friedman, S. and C. Casriel. 1988. "Drug Users' Organizations and Aids Policy." *AIDS and Public Policy Journal* 3.

Fumento, M. 1990. *The Myth of Heterosexual AIDS: How a Tragedy Has Been Distorted by the Media and Partisan Politics.* New York: Basic Books.

Gee, G. 1989. "Nurses' Attitudes and AIDS." In *Public and Professional Attitudes Toward AIDS Patients,* edited by D. Rogers and E. Ginzberg. Boulder, CO: Westview Press.

Gerstley, L.J., A.I. Alterman, T.A. McLellan and G.E. Woody. 1990. "Antisocial Personality Disorder in Patient with Substance Abuse Disorders: A Problematic Diagnosis?" *American Journal of Psychiatry* 147: 173-178.

Glenn, N. 1989. "Some Limitations of Longitudinal and Cohort Designs in Social and Behavioral Research." Pp. 55-62 in *Health Services Research Methodology: A Focus on Aids* (Conference Proceedings), edited by L. Sechrest, H. Freeman and A. Mulley. Rockville, MD: National Center for Health Services Research.

Goffman, E. 1963. *Stigma: Notes on the Management of Spoiled Identity.* Englewood Cliffs, NJ: Prentice-Hall.

Goldsmith, M. 1991. "A Sticky Issue: HIV and the IVDU." *Journal of the American Medical Association* 266(8): 1053-1054.

Herek, G. and E. Glunt. 1988. "An Epidemic of Stigma." *American Psychologist* (November): 886-890.

Kaplan, H. R. Johnson, C. Bailey and W. Simon. 1987. "The Sociological Study of AIDS: A Critical Review of the Literature and Suggested Research Agenda." *Journal of Health and Social Behavior* 28: 140-157.

Kowalewski, M. 1988. "Double Stigma and Boundary Maintenance." *Journal of Contemporary Ethnography* 17(2): 211-228.

Lindesmith, A.R. 1968. *Addiction and Opiates.* Chicago: Aldine.

Macklin, E. 1988. "AIDS: Implications for Families." *Family Relations* 37: 141-149.

Martin, E. and J. Martin. 1978. *The Black Extended Family.* Chicago: University of Chicago Press.

McAuliffe, W. and R.A. Gordon. 1975. "Issues in Testing Lindesmith's Theory." *American Journal of Sociology* 81: 154-163.

O'Donnell, T.G., et al. 1990. "Parents as Caregivers: When a Son Has Aids." *Journal of Psychosocial Nursing and Mental Health Services* 28(6): 14-7.

Poirier, R. 1988. "AIDS and Traditions of Homophobia." *Social Research* 55(3): 461-475.

Rounsaville, B.J. and H.D. Kleber. 1985. "Untreated Opiate Addicts: How Do They Differ from Those Seeking Treatment." *Archives of General Psychiatry* 42: 1072.

Rounsaville, B.J., M.M. Weissman, H. Kleber, and C. Wilber 1982. "Heterogeneity of Psychiatric Diagnosis in Treated Opiate Addicts." *Archives of General Psychiatry* 39: 16116-6.

Schwartz, R. 1989. "Physicians' Attitudes Toward AIDS." In *Public and Professional Attitudes Toward AIDS Patients,* edited by D. Rogers and E. Ginzberg. Boulder, CO: Westview Press.

Scitovsky, A.A., M. Cline, and P.R. Lee. 1986. "Medical Care Costs of Patients with Aids in San Francisco." *Journal of the American Medical Association* 256: 3103-3106.

Smith, M.D. 1989. "AIDS, IV Drug Users, and Minorities: Health Care Financing Issues." In *AIDS and Intravenous Drug Abuse Among Minorities.* National Institute of Drug Abuse. DHHS Publication No. (ADM) 90-1637. Washington, DC: U.S. Government Printing Office.

Sontag, S. 1989. *AIDS and Its Metaphors.* New York: Farrar, Straus and Giroux.
Stack, C. 1974. *All Our Kin: Strategies for Survival in a Black Community.* New York: Harper & Row.
Stein, M.D., J. Piette, V. Mor, T.J. Wachtel, J. Fleishman, K.H. Mayer, and C. Carpenter. 1991. "Differences in Access to Zidovudine (AZT) Among Symptomatic HIV-Infected Persons." *Journal of General Internal Medicine* 6(January): 35-40.
Stephens, R.C. 1991. *The Street Addict Role: A Theory of Heroin Addiction.* Albany: State University of New York Press.
Tenneriello, L., et al. 1988. "A Hospital Based Program Utilizing Methadone Patients and Others to Provide Support to Inner-city AIDS Patients." *AIDS and Public Policy Journal* 3: 67-70.
Watters, J. 1989. "Observations on the Importance of Social Context in HIV Transmission Among Intravenous Drug Users." *Journal of Drug Issues* 19(1): 9-26.
Youngstrom, N. 1991. "Antisocial Personalities Heighten Risk of AIDS." *American Psychological Association Monitor* 22(4): 23.

PROMOTING WHOSE HEALTH?
MODELS OF HEALTH PROMOTION AND
EDUCATION ABOUT HIV DISEASE

Peter Aggleton

ABSTRACT

This paper discusses the nature and value of models of health promotion as a prelude to a description of four influential models which have been used in HIV/AIDS work: the information-giving model, the self-empowerment model, the community-oriented model and the socially transformatory model. It provides illustration of each of these models in practice and discusses their strengths and limitations. Few approaches it seems are capable of realizing clear-cut, determinable outcomes. This poses major challenges for those working to prevent new cases of HIV infection and to support those already affected.

The Social and Behavioral Aspects of AIDS.
Advances in Medical Sociology, Volume 3, pages 185-200.

INTRODUCTION

It has become almost a cliché to claim that in the absence of a vaccine or cure for HIV disease, health education and health promotion are the only means of significantly affecting the course of the epidemic. But to make such a statement is to misunderstand the variety of efforts currently underway to prevent further infection and to promote the health and well-being of those already living with HIV disease. For health promotion is not a unitary concept, a "thing" that can be done, or a "process" whose effectiveness is determined solely by the technical competence of the practitioner. Neither does it occur within a social vacuum, or in contexts unsullied by divisive ideologies and the social structures that underpin them. Instead, there exist many views about how HIV/AIDS health promotion should take place and the goals that should be aimed for, as well as the means by which these can be achieved.

This paper will discuss some of the options open to those involved in HIV/AIDS health promotion, drawing upon recent experience in North America, Europe and Australasia. The aim here is to discuss some well-documented strategies which have been used in urban settings. This is not to argue that work in other contexts is somehow less important. It is, however, to recognize that a number of initiatives have been undertaken in these circumstances, work from which others can learn.

CONTEXT

HIV/AIDS health promotion is always context-bound, taking place within discrete communities and in specific settings. The impact of health promotion messages and activities is always contingent, being mediated by social expectations, popular prejudices, and group norms. These can significantly disorient the work of health promoters, and frequently produce outcomes other than those that were aimed for. An understanding of social context is therefore essential when it comes to making sense of the varying ways in which people respond to health promotion interventions. More specifically, if the strengths and limitations of contemporary styles of HIV/AIDS health promotion are to be understood, it is essential to take the following three factors into account.

First, in Europe, North America, and much of Australasia, HIV/AIDS health promotion is likely to take place in the context of widespread *heterosexual complacency,* a complacency which occasionally verges on denial. Heterosexual men, in particular, have been slow to use safer sex and for many heterosexuals, "playing safe" simply involves being more selective in the choice of prospective sexual partners. While condom sales have increased in many countries, we know little about the consistency with which they are used by heterosexual adults, nor indeed about the extent to which this increase in sales is attributable to purchasing by heterosexuals rather than gay men.

Second, HIV/AIDS health promotion takes place in the context of continued and pervasive *discrimination and prejudice.* For all the liberalism of physicians who talk about the excellent relationships they have with the "gay community," while elsewhere ruminating about what they call relapse; for all the sanctimony of health-service managers who talk glowingly of the contribution gay men as volunteers have made to community care, while elsewhere cutting statutory services; and for all the hypocrisy of health educators themselves who invite people with HIV disease to disclose their most intimate feelings and desires before audiences of a hundred or more, while elsewhere putting key resources into projects quite unrelated to these expressed needs; is as nothing compared with the more blatant prejudices and discriminatory intent still to be witnessed in the media, at home, and at work.[1]

Third it is now accepted that, even within those communities that first pioneered safer sex and first adopted safer injecting practices, behavior change has been uneven (Cohen 1991; Donoghoe, Dolan, Jones, and Stimson 1990; Stimson, Lart, Dolan, and Donoghoe 1991). In one sense, this is not at all unanticipated. Who, for example, would have expected *all* those at risk of lung cancer from cigarettes to give up smoking instantly? And who, in all seriousness, would have expected all heterosexual men, recognizing the link between unprotected penetrative sex and cervical cancer, to immediately change their behavior? While there is much to learn from the efforts of gay men who literally invented safer sex (Callen 1983) and drugs workers who won, by logical argument, the case in favor of needle and syringe exchange (Hart 1990), we still know little about how to bring about behavior change in circumstances where power relationships (of age, of patriarchy and of class) militate against the adoption of safer behaviors, and in situations where the emphasis is on sustaining rather than bringing about behavior change. Important challenges therefore remain for HIV/AIDS health promotion.

MODELS OF HEALTH PROMOTION

For several years, health promoters have been discussing the value of models of health promotion. Some have done so out of the belief that they may systematize, clarify, and make more public the different strategies that can be used to alleviate disease and illness and to promote health and well-being. Others have done so in the hope that models of health promotion may provide a means whereby to evaluate more carefully work undertaken (Aggleton 1989). Yet others have been critical of the value of models of health promotion, especially when they mystify the everyday activities of health workers and health professionals. This paper engages with these debates in order to examine the contribution that models of health promotion can make to good HIV/ AIDS work.

Some Emergent Definitions

It is appropriate to begin by identifying what is a model of health promotion. By suitably amending the framework offered by Riehl and Roy (1980), whose work was influential in establishing the credibility and widespread acceptance of nursing models, it is possible to define a model of health promotion as a systematically constructed and logically based set of concepts which identify the essential components of health promotion, together with the theoretical basis of these components and the values required for their use by the practitioner.

There are a number of key elements within this definition. First, it is important to recognize that health promotion models are systematically constructed and developed. They are not simply a few personal opinions about how health promotion should take place. Second, many of them build upon insights derived from other disciplines and areas of study, especially those in the natural, medial, and social sciences. Models of health beliefs and health behavior, for example, are not infrequently based on insights derived from social psychology (e.g., Becker 1984; Janz and Becker 1984; Fishbein and Ajzen 1985; Tones 1987), whereas numerous assessment and planning frameworks derive from more general work within systems theory. Third, models of health promotion are not neutral; they are linked closely to views about how disease and illness might best be avoided, and about how health and well-being are best attained. In so doing, they articulate concern about the extent to which individuals, rather than the state, should be responsible for their own health. Finally, models of health promotion differ from one another in terms of the extent to which they are concerned with education *about* health, education *in relation to* health and education *for* health.

Goals and Means

In general terms, models of health promotion have something to say about the *goals* that health promoters and clients might aim for as well as the means by which these might be achieved. Thus, we can distinguish between those that have changes in knowledge, attitudes, and behavior as their goal and which advocate information giving as the means by which to achieve this, and those which aim for either self- or community-empowerment through greater individual or collective participation in health issues.

In one of the first papers to attempt a systematic analysis of different models of health education, French and Adams (1986) differentiate between three broad paradigms within which health promotion can take place—the behavior-change model, the self-empowerment model and the collective-action model. While the first of these models attempts to improve health by changing people's behavior, and the second to improve health by developing people's ability to understand and control their health status to whatever extent is possible within their environmental circumstances, the third aims to improve health by changing environmental, social, and economic factors through community involvement and action. As French and Adams (1989) subsequently acknowledge, this initial approach had several shortcomings.

For example, the first of these models is not the only one to be concerned with eliciting behavior change. This is a goal linked to many different kinds of health promotion. Further problems relate to French and Adams' characterization of the collective-action model. Some stem from the fact that the term community and hence community involvement is heavily loaded with positive connotations. So much so, that it "enjoys a halo of approval from those occupying widely divergent positions on the political and ideological spectrum"(Butcher 1986, p. 89). Thus, some of those who welcome community involvement in health issues do so out of a commitment to social justice, whereas others do so out of a concern that health care is provided in the interests of consumers, rather than the producers, of medical care (Richardson and Gray, 1987). This latter, more consumerist view can be used to legitimate competition between different communities of interest such that resources are allocated to the most vocal, the most articulate, and the most powerful, rather than those with greatest need.

More recently, French and Adams (1989) have differentiated between *community participation* as a "process (which may) bring about a planned change in community life," *community empowerment* as a "process by which health educators try to enable people to increase control or at least a sense of control over their lives and health," and *social action,* an overtly political process which involves the "forceful advocacy of a particular position in which community members are mobilized to use methods of conflict and political pressure to achieve their aims." These are helpful distinctions in that they differentiate among a variety of types of community involvement in health issues. The typology, however, still fails to distinguish as clearly as it might do between goals and means. Defined this way, community participation and social action are clearly the means by which certain goals may be achieved, whereas community empowerment would appear to be both a means and a goal, depending on the context in which it is used.

One way out of this dilemma is to examine the extent to which different community-based health promotion initiatives seek to challenge the orthodoxies and commitments of modern biomedicine—be these to do with the hierarchical relationships between practitioners and clients, the overemphasis on cure at the expense of prevention, or the individualization of responsibility for health issues. By doing this, it may be possible to differentiate between what Watt and Rodmell (1988) have characterized as supplementary and oppositional health promotion practices.

Another, more radical strategy might be to examine the extent to which community-based health promotion initiatives seek to challenge structural inequality in society—in particular, inequalities of class, gender, sexuality, ethnicity, and culture. Such an approach must involve a consideration of *outcomes* as well as goals and intentions, for if resistance theory has taught us anything, it is that the most radical initiatives can sometimes have the most conservative effects.[2] Only when health promotion succeeds in realizing social change can we talk about the intervention having been genuinely *socially transformatory*. Otherwise, we might better talk merely of there having been a *community-oriented* intervention, one which may hold the potential to bring about social change, but which may or may not realize this.

It would be nice to be able to transcend all of these dilemmas by moving beyond the partial typology of styles of health promotion which presently exists. But to do without considering concrete instances of health promotion in general and HIV/AIDS health promotion in particular would be to run the risk of academicizing what are essentially practical concerns. For it is only *in practice* that we can identify the main features of different strategies and approaches, and it is only *through practice* that we can enable people to respond to the health challenges that confront them.

Four Models of HIV/AIDS Promotion

This concern with practice has led to the identification of four key models of health promotion influential in HIV/AIDS work—the information-giving approach, the self-empowerment approach, the community-oriented approach, and the socially transformatory approach (Aggleton and Homans 1987; Aggleton 1989). In the original formulation, these models were differentiated in terms of the goals they set for health promotion and the means by which these might be achieved. Taking on board the distinction made earlier between intentions and outcomes, it might be better to characterize them now in terms of the goals they specify, the means they advocate, and the *outcomes* they seem capable of realizing (see Table 1).

The first and second of these models will of course be familiar to many health educators since they constitute the dominant paradigms within which much *official* and *alternative* health promotion takes place. The third and fourth models need some clarification however, both conceptually and in relation to work in the HIV/AIDS field. Community-oriented approaches move away from the idea that individuals should be responsible for their own health. They suggest instead that people should collectively identify and act upon the factors which affect their health and well-being. Such models range from those concerned with self-help, through those which involve participation in community health groups, to those which adopt a community development approach (Watt and Rodmell 1988). The outcomes of community-oriented

Table 1.   Four Models of HIV/AIDS Health Promotion

Model	Goals	Means	Likely Outcomes
Information-giving	To enhance knowledge modify attitudes, and change behavior.	Provision of information in talks, videos, films and so forth.	Improved knowledge levels. Little change in attitudes and behavior.
Self-empowerment	To enhance the ability to act in a considered way, not on the basis of emotional reactions.	Small-group work. Values clarification. Assertiveness training.	An enhanced sense of self-efficacy and personal well-being (both may fade with time).
Community-oriented	To enhance the ability to act in a considered way, not on the basis of emotional reactions.	Small group work. Outreach work. Community attachment work.	Enhanced community participation and involvement with conservative, liberal, and radical effects.
Socially transformatory	To bring about far-reaching social change so as to remedy health inequalities.	Small and then larger-group work to develop critical insight and to act on the basis of this.	Radically diminished levels of health inequality. Eradication of divisive and oppressive ideololgies.

initiatives cannot, however, be predicted in advance. Some may be liberating and supportive, whereas others may be containing and oppressive. There is no reason whatsoever to suppose that community-oriented styles of health promotion per se bring about social and economic change. Nor can they guarantee enhanced levels of social justice. Their effects are contingent upon the political projects of those who use this style of health promotion and the context within which they take place.

Socially transformative approaches, on the other hand, are self-consciously committed to bringing about social change. All are likely to be community based to the extent that they involve collectivities of individuals, but only a few are likely to lay the foundations for far-reaching social change. Socially transformatory health promotion, too, may have uneven and unpredictable effects. It may reinforce dominant ideologies and social divisions or it may challenge them and, like any other kind of health promotion, its short-term effects may differ from those achieved over a longer period of time. These tensions are something that health educators committed to this kind of approach have constantly to struggle with if their projects are to bring about desired goals and outcomes.

Table 2. A Partially Constructed Matrix of Communication Possibilities Within an Information-Giving Approach

				Modality			
Context	One-to-one	Small Group	Mass Media	Local Media	Small Media	Out-reach/ Detached Work	Lecture/Film/Video
Professional work-related	Employment-related counseling.	Values clarification work. Skills training.					Large-scale information-giving.
Personal	Pre-/and post-test counseling.		Awareness raising.	Using a local radio station to advertise a local AIDS line.	Using lapel badges to reinforce key messages.	Educating "hard-to-reach" groups.	

Information Giving

Information giving is the strategy most frequently adopted by central and local governments, health authorities, and non-governmental organizations involved in HIV/AIDS work. In order to characterize the many ways in which information giving can take place, it is useful to distinguish between *modality* and *context*. By modality is meant the means by which information is imparted—be it on a one-to-one basis by word of mouth, over a telephone hot-line, by small-group work, via the mass media, via outreach or detached work, or through local or small media. The term context, on the other hand, distinguishes between occasions where the emphasis is on meeting professional needs and those where personal concerns are more paramount. Those two principles can be used to constitute a matrix of communication possibilities of use to health promoters who desire to be more inclusive in the strategies they adopt (see Table 2).

In the early days of the epidemic, much emphasis was given to the provision of medical and scientific information whereby people might protect themselves and others from infection. The first U.K. public information initiative, for example, launched in 1986, talked glibly of "T-Helper Cells" and "rectal sex" to an audience well versed neither in the niceties of the immune system nor in the anatomy of the gastrointestinal tract (Department of Health and Social Security 1987). Not infrequently, moreover, such information has been linked to overtly moral agendas promoting chastity before marriage and fidelity within it, and denying the "authenticity" of anything other than penetrative vaginal sex (Homans and Aggleton 1988).

Information-giving strategies can also be used to establish the climate within which other interventions can take place, as well as to consolidate community work already undertaken (Valdiserri 1989). Thus, the 1990 Australian National AIDS Education Campaign for gay and bisexual men aimed to build upon community and grass-roots work already carried out by local AIDS Councils. Its emphasis was on sustaining behavior change in circumstances where desire and intimacy may interfere with the practice of safer sex. These include relationships where both partners may be HIV antibody positive and relationships where a developing level of commitment and trust may encourage one or both parties not to practice safer sex (Commonwealth Department of Community Services and Health 1990).

In other information giving-approaches, however, there continues to be much talk of "catching" AIDS and "avoiding" it, almost as if a simple social algebra needs only be invoked to reduce the risk. More recently too, there is increasing debate about how to access the "hard to reach"—those whose lives do not bring them into contact with the health promotion messages offered by physicians, health education officers, teachers, and others. What such approaches often fail to recognize is the limited value of health promotion strategies which fail to engage in any meaningful way with people's fears and anxieties, with complex processes of social and personal denial, and with the structural forces that may prevent women, for example, from "insisting" that their male partners use a condom and younger people from acquiring and practicing the skills whereby to negotiate and enjoy safer sex (Holland, Ramazanoglu, Scott, Sharpe, and Thompson 1991).

Self-empowerment

In contrast to health promotion strategies which seek to provide information in order to bring about behavior change are those which recognize that values, attitudes and emotions may affect a person's ability to act in a considered way. Using participatory forms of eduction and small group work, such techniques aim to *empower* individuals in their relationships with others. Three main approaches can be distinguished: those based on principles derived from one-to-one client-centered counseling, those that advocate participation in group-based activities and role play, and those that promote individual participation in emergent community organizations and structures. Some self-empowerment strategies aim to foster enhanced self-esteem and personal growth, others aim to help clients be more assertive, most usually within the context of negotiating for safer sex.

Some self-empowerment approaches draw upon prior experience in women's health, and a few move beyond the individual to engage with broader issues such as social expectations, roles in society, peer pressures, and conformity. What all emphasize, however, is that the solution for many HIV/AIDS related problems and difficulties lies within the *individual*. With the right opportunities, individuals may acquire the self-awareness and the skills to transform their relationships and their lives more generally.

There is now clear evidence to suggest that, in comparison to more didactic methods, self-empowerment approaches can be more effective in bringing about attitudinal if not behavioral change. Early work on the San Francisco Stop AIDS project, for example, whose aim was to engender a personal commitment to safer sex behavior, suggested that well-facilitated group activities could bring about changes in attitudes (Puckett and Bye 1987), a finding subsequently confirmed in Miller, Booraem, Flowers, and Inverson's (1990) field-based evaluation of this particular approach. In a more directly comparative study, Leviton et al. (1990) examined the medium- and longer-term consequences for gay men of participating either in a 60-90 minute formal educational session or in such a session followed by group work and role play examining attitudes and feelings about safer sex. They found that the latter condition was much more effective in promoting positive attitudes toward aspects of safer sex such as condom use.[3]

The individualism of self-empowerment approaches has, however, been criticised, as has their relative neglect of the economic, cultural, and sexual forces which structure or pattern social relationships. It is not unknown, for example, for participants to leave an HIV/AIDS health promotion workshop feeling more empowered, but for these same feelings to fade rapidly thereafter. Concerns such as these, which can be very real at the time, are taken up by some community-oriented initiatives.

Community-oriented Approaches

Community-oriented health promotion starts from the premise that it is important for people to act collectively around shared interests in relation to health. That said, the term itself encompasses a range of very different health education activities, varying from those that take place *within* a community, through those which take place *for* a community, to those which more explicitly aim to *develop* a community. These distinctions are crucial when it comes to understanding the strengths and limitations of this kind of work. Not all community-based work will lead to community development, only that which self-consciously has this as a goal is likely to succeed, and even here the outcomes are far from predictable. For example, health promotion initiatives imposed on a community from outside may be perceived as threatening or even patronizing, and in the medium- to long-term such top-down strategies may prove less effective than those which originate from the expressed needs of communities themselves (Beattie 1987).

An illustration of this latter approach is offered by the Toehold initiative in Queensland, Australia. This sought to recruit younger gay men to a community-based, peer-led HIV/AIDS education project. Publicity for the project, in the form of an introduction card distributed at gay community events, was generated by an existing gay youth group which served thereafter as a base for activities such as discussion groups (Davis 1990). While activity such as this is notoriously difficult to sustain, and while the goals pursued may be very different from those originally anticipated, such programs play a vital role in developing networks of community support which outlive the interventions themselves.

The work of this particular project, however, highlights an important factor to be borne in mind when thinking about community-oriented HIV/AIDS health promotion. The communities within which interventions take place are not homogenous, but culturally and socially fragmented—by age, by class, by culture, and in some cases by gender. This renders any simple notion of community development problematic. It is, for example, absurd to talk about carrying out HIV/AIDS health promotion within the "injecting drug user community" within the "gay community," or even worse, within the "heterosexual community," for these communities as homogeneous and unified entities do not exist. Admittedly, there may be more of a common identity and common purpose among those such as gay men and injecting drug users, who have experienced stigmatization, oppression, and discrimination, but there is diversity here too—diversity of need, diversity of expression, and diversity of desire. This heterogeneity may account for the lack of success many interventions have had in reaching minority ethnic communities, and calls for more culturally appropriate responses (De la Cancela 1989).

It may also explain why some of the most successful community-oriented initiatives have adopted a dynamic and *socially differentiated* approach by responding to the expressed needs of different groups, and modifying their approach over time. Thus, community-oriented safer sex work at the Gay Men's Health Crisis (GMHC) in New York has passed through a number of phases. Initially, the emphasis was on "Eroticizing Safer Sex" workshops to inform men that certain behaviors were life threatening and to help men change from high-risk to lower-risk behaviors (Palacios-Jiminez and Shernoff 1988). Subsequently, and as a response to changing needs, other activities have been developed. These include "Men Meeting Men" workshops in which the emphasis is on coping, support, dating, the sharing of feelings, and sexual intimacy. More recently, a third style of workshop has been introduced—titled "Sex, Dating and Intimacy in the Age of AIDS"—which aims to enhance self-esteem, sustain safer sex, provide support for those beginning new relationships, and strengthen participants' involvement in gay social networks (Shernoff and Bloom 1991).

In the above sequence of events, we can witness a transition from interventions *within* and *for* the community, to those that more explicitly seek to *develop* it. By strengthening the bonds between individuals, safer-sex events such as these hold the potential to enhance self-esteem and consolidate community identification. By so doing, some may lay the foundations for more socially transformatory projects and for community activism around HIV/AIDS and allied issues.

Socially Transformatory Approaches

In a recent article, Altman (1990) has drawn attention to some of the challenges presently confronting community-based AIDS organizations and AIDS service Organizations. These include questions about aims, purposes, and structure; about the constituencies whose interests they claim to represent; and about the relationships that should be cultivated with sponsors and funding bodies. Simultaneously, there has been growing recognition that if community-oriented HIV/AIDS health promotion is to have lasting effectiveness, it must be linked to changes in policy and legislation. As Silin (1987, p. 36) states:

While we can each play a role in ending the epidemic by practicing safer sex, as a community we must also learn to fight for funding, legal protection and attitudinal transformation necessary to ensure our future survival.

Together these twin sources of impetus have encouraged some HIV/AIDS educators and community workers to be more proactive in their role, and to advocate more direct means of bringing about social change. Some have found scope for their activism in groups such as ACTUP (AIDS Coalition to Unleash Power) whereas others have chosen to work in a more mainstream way within existing structures, using established procedures and protocols.

Stimulated by a concern to change not only the priorities of politicians, resource managers, and decision makers, but also the social relations of HIV/AIDS (between doctors and "patients," between "experts" and "lay people," between "us" and "them"), ACTUP came together in New York in early 1987 as a diverse nonpartisan movement committed to direct action. Its aims were to change the priorities of politicians, to make treatment drugs more accessible, and to draw attention to government intransigence and inactivity in the face of a major epidemic. Drawing upon long-standing U.S. traditions of civil disobedience in order to secure fundamental human rights, ACTUP has staged protests in locations as diverse as the Golden Gate Bridge (January 1989), Burroughs Wellcome's offices (April 1989), the New York Stock Exchange (September 1989) and the U.S. National Institutes of Health (May 1990) (Walter 1990). The actions of local ACTUP groups in the United States have since been emulated elsewhere in the world (Goddard 1990).

The success of such groups in challenging dominant agendas around HIV/AIDS cannot be disputed, and the opening up of access to experimental treatment drugs in the United States and elsewhere is largely a consequence of their actions. This success is attributable to at least three qualities—the use of research and other "hard evidence" to justify the claims and demands they make; the creative use of media such as leaflets, street boards, film, and video; and the successful channeling of anger, energy, and frustration into a grass-roots movement for social change (Ariss 1990). Concurrently there has emerged a new social identity—the AIDS activist—the person committed to tackling the epidemic through direct action so as to bring about far-reaching social change.

More recently, however, such organizations have been subject to internal fragmentation and division, with some members arguing for closer links to other civil rights organizations, such as those working against sexism and racism, and others arguing for a narrower charter, one focusing specifically on issues to do with HIV/AIDS (Gallagher 1991). In part, such conflict may be attributable to the diversity of their original membership, but it raises important questions about the extent to which work around HIV/AIDS should be linked to other agendas, particularly those that would have us understand health inequalities in broader structural terms.

CONCLUSIONS

When work on models of health promotion first began, the aim was to clarify what health education and health promotion might be about. The advent of HIV disease, an incurable and potentially life-threatening condition affecting millions of people worldwide, has added new impetus to this project, not least because of the need to learn from past experiences and to develop innovatory and effective responses. While it has often been seen as important to differentiate between goals and means in health promotion, from the initiatives examined here it is clear that *outcomes* are a third set of factors that need to be taken into account when analyzing and evaluating the strengths and weaknesses of different approaches.

If future work is to bear dividends, it will need to examine more closely the interplay between goals, means, contexts, and outcomes, for it is only by doing this that we can fully comprehend why some projects come to fruition and others do not. This is not to suggest that, with the right combination of factors, an intervention will inevitably succeed. Rather, it is to argue for an analysis of the complex ways in which environmental, social, political, economic, and ideological circumstances can disorient, build on, reinforce, or limit the effectiveness of HIV/AIDS health promotion. Clearly, there is much that remains to be done, but with the necessary effort, will, and political commitment, the task can be accomplished.

ACKNOWLEDGMENTS

I would like to thank Simon Watney, Meurig Horton, and Gary Dowsett who have been continuing sources of inspiration; Ian Warwick and Stuart Watson for keeping me sane in moments of great stress; and colleagues in the Health and Education Research Unit at Goldsmiths' College, University of London for their commitment, humor and enduring support.

NOTES

1.   While this is not the place in which to document such responses, which has been amply done already (see, for example, Watney 1987; Wellings 1988; Clift, and Stears, Legg, Memon,and Ryan 1990), it is the place to emphasize that contrary to popular belief, discrimination and prejudice have not disappeared.

2.   See, for example, the work of Giroux (1983) in the field of education.

3.   See also Valdiserri et al. (1987).

REFERENCES

Aggleton, P.J. 1989. "Evaluating AIDS Education". Pp. 220-237 in *AIDS: Social Representations, Social Practices,* edited by P.J. Aggleton, P. Davies, and G. Hart. Lewes, UK: Falmer Press.

Aggleton, P.J. and H. Homans. 1987. *Educating about AIDS: A Discussion Document for Community Physicians, Health Education Officers and others with a Responsibility for Education about HIV Infection and AIDS.* Bristol, UK: National Health Service Training Authority.

Altman, D. 1990. "Community-Based Organisations and the Future". *Australian National AIDS Bulletin* 4(1): 12-14.

Ariss, R. 1990. "Acting Up in America". *Australian National AIDS Bulletin* 4(8): 12-14.

Beattie, A. 1987. "Community Development for Health: From Practice to Theory?" *Radical Health Promotion* 4: 12-18.

Becker, M.H. 1984. *The Health Belief Model and Personal Health Behavior.* New Jersey; Charles B. Slack.

Butcher, H. 1986. "The 'Community Practice' Approach to Local Service Provision: An Analysis of Recent Developments". *Community Development Journal* 21(2): 88-100.

Callen, M. 1983. *How to Have Sex in an Epidemic.* New York: News from the Front Publications.

Clift, S., D. Stears, S. Legg, A. Memon, and L. Ryan. 1990. "Blame and Young People's Moral Judgements about AIDS". Pp. 53-72 in *AIDS: Individual, Cultural and Policy Dimensions,* edited by P.J. Aggleton, P. Davies and G. Hart. Basingstoke, UK: Falmer Press.

Cohen, M. 1991. "Changing to Safer Sex: Personality, Logic and Habit." Pp. 19-43 in *AIDS: Responses, Interventions and Care,* edited by P.J. Aggleton, P. Davies and G. Hart. London: Falmer Press.

Commonwealth Department of Community Services and Health. 1990. "A National Campaign for Gay and Bisexual Men." *Australian AIDS Bulletin* 5(1): 26-27.

Davis, M. 1990 "Peer Education and a Framework for Change in Queensland." *Australian National AIDS Bulletin* 4(7): 37-40.

De la Cancela, V. 1989. "Minority AIDS Prevention: Moving Beyond Cultural Perspectives Towards Sociological Empowerment." *AIDS Education and Prevention* 1(2): 141-153.

Donoghoe, M., K. Dolan, S. Jones, and G.V. Stimson. 1990. "National Syringe Exchange Monitoring Study: An Interim Report." Report to the Department of Health, London. Charing Cross and Westminster Medical School, Centre for Research on Drugs and Health Behavior.

Fishbein, M. and I. Ajzen. 1985. *Belief, Attitude, Intention and Behavior: An Introduction to Theory and Research.* Reading, MA: Addison-Wesley.

French, J. and L. Adams. 1986. "From Analysis to Synthesis." *Health Education Journal* 45(2): 71-4.

French, J. and L. Adams. 1989. "An Overview of Current Models of Health Promotion." Paper presented at the Health for Who? Symposium, Public Health Alliance/Society of Health Education and Health Promotion Officers, London.

Gallagher, J. 1991. "Oregon Activists Split over Sexism Charges: Lawsuits Threatened." *The Advocate,* (March 26), p. 24.

Goddard, M. 1990. "No More Mister Nice Guys." *Australian National AIDS Bulletin* 4(5): 7-12.

Hart, G. 1990. "Needle Exchange in Historical Context: Responses to the 'Drugs Problem.' " Pp. 133-142 in *AIDS: Individual, Cultural and Policy Dimensions,* edited by P.J. Aggleton, P. Davies, and G. Hart. Basingstoke, UK: Falmer Press.

Holland, J., C. Ramazanoglu, S. Scott, S. Sharpe, and R. Thompson. 1991. "Between Embarrassment and Trust: Young Women and the Diversity of Condom Use." Pp. 127-

149 in *AIDS: Responses, Interventions and Care,* edited by P.J. Aggleton, P. Davies, and G. Hart. London: Falmer Press.

Homans, H. and P.J. Aggleton. 1988. "Health Education, HIV Infection and AIDS." Pp. 154-176 in *Social Aspects of AIDS,* edited by P.J. Aggleton and H. Homans. Lewes, UK: Falmer Press.

Janz, J.K. and M.H. Becker. 1984. "The Health Belief Model: A Decade Later." *Health Education Quarterly* 11: 47.

Leviton, L., R. Valdiserri, D. Lyter, C. Callaghan, L. Kingsley, J. Huggins, and C. Rinaldo. 1990. "Preventing HIV Infection in Gay and Bisexual Men: Experimental Evaluation of Attitude Change from Two Risk Reduction Interventions." *AIDS Education and Prevention* 2(2): 95-108.

Miller, T., C. Booraem, J.V. Flowers, and A. Iverson. 1990. "Changes in Knowledge, Attitudes and behavior as a Result of a Community-Based AIDS Prevention Programme." *AIDS Education and Prevention* 2(1): 12-23.

Palacios-Jiminez, L. and M. Shernoff. 1988. "AIDS: Prevention is the only Vaccine Available: An AIDS Prevention Education Programme." *Journal of Social Work and Human Sexuality* 6(2): 135-150.

Puckett, S. and L. Bye. 1987. *The Stop AIDS Project: An Interpersonal AIDS Prevention Programme.* San Francisco, CA: The Stop AIDS Project Inc.

Richardson, A. and C. Gray. 1987. *Promoting Health Through Participation.* London: Policy Studies Institute.

Riehl, J. and C. Roy. 1980. *Conceptual Models for Nursing Practice.* 2nd ed. Norwalk, CT: Appleton-Century-Crofts.

Shernoff, M. and D. Bloom. 1991. "Designing Effective AIDS Prevention Workshops for Gay and Bisexual Men." *AIDS Education and Prevention* 3(1): 31-46.

Silin, J. 1987. "Dangerous Knowledge." *Christopher Street* 113: 34-40.

Stimson, G., R. Lart, K. Dolan, and M. Donoghoe. 1991. "The Future of Syringe Exchange in the Public Health Prevention of HIV Infection." Pp. 225-233 in *AIDS: Responses, Interventions and Care,* edited by P.J. Aggleton, P. Davies, and G. Hart. London: Falmer Press.

Tones, K. 1987. "Health Promotion, Affective Education and the Personal-Social Development of Young People." Pp. 3-44 in edited by K. David and T. Williams. *Health Education in Schools,* 2nd ed. London: Harper and Row.

Valdiserri, R.O. 1989. *Preventing AIDS.* New Brunswick, NJ: Rutgers University Press.

Department of Health and Social Security. 1987. *AIDS: Monitoring Responses to the Public Educati on Campaign, 1986-1987.* London: Her Majesty's Stationery Office.

Valdiserri, R.O., D. Lyter, L. Kingsley, L. Leviton, J. Schofield, J. Huggins, M. Ho, and C. Ronaldo. 1987. "The Effect of Group Education on Improving Attitudes about AIDS Risk Reduction." *New York State Journal of Medicine* (May): 272-279.

Walter, D. 1990. "Does Civil Disobedience Still Work?" *The Advocate* (November 20), 34-38.

Watney, S. 1987. *Policing Desire: Pornography, AIDS and the Media.* London: Comedia/Methuen.

Watt, A. and S. Rodmell. 1988. *The Politics of Health Education.* London: Routledge & Kegan Paul.

Wellings, K. 1988. "Perceptions of Risk—Media Treatments of AIDS." Pp. 83-105 in *Social Aspects of AIDS,* edited by P.J. Aggleton and H. Homans. Lewes, UK: Falmer Press.

THE SOCIOLOGICAL IMAGINATION IN AIDS PREVENTION EDUCATION AMONG GAY MEN

Philip M. Kayal

ABSTRACT

"Safer-sex" education in AIDS prevention programs is often grounded in a systematic set of social-order theories reflecting heterosexist or homophobic views of gay male sexuality. These programs also reveal the ideologies of their planners and funding sources by assuming that homosexual behavior is essentially impersonal and promiscuous and that unsafe sexual behavior is rooted in ignorance and psychological "compulsivity." If unsafe sex among gays is considered a social problem, rather than an individual failure, then prevention programs that begin with psychological premises are inappropriate. They leave institutionalized and internalized homophobia (the structural sources of maladaptive behavior) unchallenged. This paper compares psychologically oriented behavioral modification as a strategy of change with communal empowerment as an alternate antidote to unsafe sex. In the tradition of the "sociological imagination," the solution to a social problem (like HIV

The Social and Behavioral Aspects of AIDS.
Advances in Medical Sociology, Volume 3, pages 201-221.
Copyright © 1993 by JAI Press Inc.
All Rights of reproduction in any form reserved.
ISBN: 1-55938-439-5

transmission) is in the political process. Effective social change commences with the establishment of community (a political act) and, in AIDS prevention, the individual and collective interests must first be joined to prevent mutual annihilation.

INTRODUCTION

In 1985, because of the imminent threat that AIDS posed to the survival of the gay community, Gay Men's Health Crisis (GMHC), an AIDS-specific social service agency in New York City, pioneered the development of an AIDS prevention education program known as The 800 Men Project. It was designed to address the sexual transmission of the disease, at least among gay men. Being the first and foremost mobilization against AIDS in the United States, GMHC was under pressure to do something immediately practical about AIDS. With its national reputation for service delivery and its expertise in AIDS policy development well-established (Kobasa 1990), its new program became a model for other cities confronting the heavy burden of AIDS and was opened in time to thousands of others beyond the original 800 men who had participated in the first trial sessions.

This paper examines the ideological roots of The 800 Men Project, with an eye toward determining how a psychological approach to the problem of HIV transmission affects not only the allocation of responsibility in AIDS prevention, but the potential for community empowerment, an alternate strategy. By sociologically assessing the assumptions and methods of GMHC's program, a different, albeit political, solution to the dangerous spread of AIDS through sexual contact will be identified. Like all social problems (Mills 1959), the fulmination of HIV is ultimately rooted in social arrangements which work against self and communal actualization, leaving people guilt-ridden, hence self-destructive.

For gays, prejudiced social arrangements create powerless "others" and "outsiders." In this state of emanation (Halpern 1969), impersonal maladaptive sexual and social behavior becomes normative and, in the context of AIDS, is manifested in disassociation from community or the practice of unsafe-sex. Conversely, self-acceptance is measured by identification with the life and problems of the community and collectively becoming sexually responsible. By joining the individual and collective interest (Abalos 1986), the gay community can politically undermine the existing social order and those legitimating ideologies which foster destructive behavior. This application of the "sociological imagination" to AIDS prevention will focus on the links between people and their relationship as a community to the broader society.

ABOUT GMHC AND THE 800 MEN PROJECT

Though community-owned and gay identified, GMHC services are used without charge by nearly 40 percent of all people with AIDS (PWAs) in New

York, regardless of race, gender, or sexual orientation. As an alternative community-based initiative (Rothschild-Witt 1979) committed to protecting and preserving a collective gay life and identity, GMHC had to take up the cause of AIDS prevention through education about its transmission (Shilts 1987). There was enormous need and its accepted credibility would have faltered if it didn't sponsor a program which would both celebrate homosexuality and yet save lives.[1]

However, by narrowly defining the need for AIDS prevention primarily in terms of "safer-sex" techniques for gay men, The 800 Men Project virtually excluded all other at-risk populations. GMHC could, thus, stick quite close to the stereotypical understanding of homosexuals as preeminently and definably sexual actors (Greenberg 1988). GMHC smartly reinforced the impression that it was in tune with "popular" gay needs and on target about how the question of AIDS prevention should be defined and its sexual transmission reduced. While it stressed information as the best antidote to both gay and AIDS hysteria, its accent on safer-sex practices was not as free of ideological and outside constraints as generally believed.

Because it is rooted in time and place, GMHC primarily encourages behavioral modification, but only in a way which maintains an older, more familiar sexual and interactive script as encapsulated in the gay clone outlined by Levine (1979). Though commonplace and popular as sexual behaviors, or postures, the project assumes that dysfunctional gay male sexual behavior, even if done safely, need not itself be assessed. It also assumes that impersonal "lone ranger" sex can be made safer through information and erotic "resocialization."[2]

Tailoring a service and education program to gay needs is necessary for no other reason than GMHC's name (identity) and the fact that it depends on the gay community for volunteers, staff, clients, and 75 percent of its financial support (Gay Men's Health Crisis 1989). Unlike GMHC, however, PWAs come from diverse populations, reflecting the fact that AIDS disproportionately affects, in ever-increasing numbers, poor Latinos, blacks, and drug users and their sexual partners (Friedman et al. 1987). At GMHC, all of these populations are difficult to reach for sociocultural and historical reasons (Marin and Marin 1990),[3] not the least of which are the gay stigma attached to AIDS, homophobia, at least in some quarters of the African-American population (Hammonds 1987), and the prevalence of IV drug-abuse as a mode of transmission among minorities.[4]

There is also a political economy behind the decision to concentrate on gay male sexual behavior besides GMHC's "elegant" and gay corporate culture and the pressures generated on it by its own large bureaucracy. The 800 Men Project supports social expectations as attached to governmental funding requirements and ideological beliefs about the location of social pathology in the psychology of individuals rather than in social arrangements, like discrimination and homophobia—the inordinate fear and loathing of homosexuals and homosexuality (Weinberg 1973).

Though these dehumanizing structural realities surround everyday gay life and explain why both AIDS and unsafe sex are significant social and political issues, they are generally ignored in AIDS prevention programs. Though it needs to be addressed as such, safer-sex education generally leaves unattended the institutionalized violence forever present against the gay psyche. The 800 Men Project, however, actually reflects dysfunctional cultural assumptions about gay life-style expectations and the meaning and place of sexual activity in identity formation.

From its inception, GMHC faced several pressing dilemmas: how to "publicize" AIDS and immediately contain its spread, how to mobilize the community to "own" the disease and begin caring for PWAs, how to help gays be healthfully sexual in an epidemic (Barnett 1986), and how to establish a new life-giving homosexual identity—in gay and heterosexual minds alike—that transcends the impersonal, patriarchal sexual behavior imposed upon gays by powerful heterosexists and their homophobic institutions (Irvine 1990). To successfully argue that AIDS is a scientific, biological, and medical problem, rather than a problem in morality, deviance (Brandt 1985; Galliher and Tyree 1985) or even homosexuality as such, GMHC could only stick to the scientific facts of sexual transmission, once these "facts" began to emerge after 1985. It would be inopportune to recognize AIDS as a collective crisis in interpersonal relations and community health.

To maintain community support, moreover, GMHC would not address "value questions," especially those which go to the core of gay identity and popular homosexual practice. Nor could GMHC question the propriety of patriarchal sexual behavior (Johnston 1979), even though it impacted negatively on the communalization process and, hence, the solution on the political level to AIDS-homophobia (the increased hatred of gays because of AIDS and the disavowal of AIDS because it is thought of as gay). In the afterglow of Stonewall (the birthplace in 1969 of the modern gay rights movement), proposing behavioral changes which appeared moralistic, condemnatory, or authoritarian (Adkins 1986a) would be distrustful, dysfunctional, and divisive. Likewise, GMHC could not appear to be advocating direct, confrontational politics over AIDS policy or be directly and publicly supportive of still-illegal activities when receiving government grants.

To get even short-term funding for prevention, GMHC programmers had to consider federal concerns about condoning homosexual behavior.[5] All that was possible in AIDS prevention, therefore, was education about transmission and treating individually "compulsive" sexual activity. If maladaptive homosexual behavior could be defined as an illness, then, at least some state funding would be made available, and even appear magnanimous. As part of its "family" agenda, the federal government wanted an end to homosexual sex in any and every fashion and hardly would support reeroticizing "deviant" sex in the interests of collective health. Hence, GMHC could and would safely advocate only behavioral modification on the subjective, psychological level. While useful in the short run, this approach decidedly depoliticizes by opposing the individual interest to the collective need.

Washington has consistently resisted any AIDS education which challenges the social environment out of which maladaptive behavior springs or which would direct human potential into community empowerment as an alternative solution to what it sees as individually self-destructive behavior. A politicizing approach would simply be too disruptive of prevailing (and religiously legitimated) social arrangements. Under pressure from Senator Jesse Helms, who saw safer-sex as advocating "safe-sodomy" (Poirier 1988), it would not allow even the use of rationalized and psychological ("therapeutic") interventions which would educate individuals about safer-sex techniques in a way which would help them to accept and practice them. In any case, no safer drug-using proposals would ever be supported and little money would be available for community health and development. This, despite the contrary public rhetoric of the last two Republican federal administrations (Palmer and Sawhill 1984; Kayal 1990a).

Things differed somewhat at the state level. The New York AIDS Institute in Albany (headed by the first executive director of GMHC) was able to allocate state money to teach grown men "how to" and "what to" erotize sexually and safely. New York State's interest was purely pragmatic and practical. AIDS was a very expensive illness and New York led the nation in the number of cases and potential fatalities. While the proposed program offered help in reducing the number of future cases, it also maintained homophobic institutional arrangements, though they impact negatively on gays and lesbians and encourage maladaptive behavior. Basically, The 800 Men Project was a "liberal" compromise with advocates of total abstinence.

PROJECT ASSUMPTIONS AND CONTENT

In the attempt to balance homosexual expression with community interests, GMHC had no choice but to define unsafe-sex as an individual pathology instead of a reflection of internalized and normative social expectations. Ideologically (and conveniently), rather than being considered a social problem, dysfunctional sexual behavior was thought a personal aberration. Given the popularity and availability of assumedly apolitical, psychological solutions to social problems, this is not surprising. However, GMHC's objective and approach both have political consequences on collective and individual well-being.

The basic assumptions underlying The 800 Men Project were that the subjectively erotic is changeable through operative conditioning and that maladaptive sexual behavior is rooted in "compulsivity" (Wedin 1984a) or the inability and unwillingness to act differently, even in a life-threatening epidemic. These traits are considered major characteristics of sexually "overactive" gay men (Quadland 1983), whether they act safely or unsafely. Defenders of sexual compulsivity (as an explanatory variable) must believe that sexual activity for pleasure is a scarce resource that should be preserved and used reservedly.

Yet, since what mattered medically was neither the quantity of partners nor the quality of interactions between them, but the specific sexual activities performed, GMHC could justify its belief that if safer sexual activities were eroticized, then, so-called compulsive gay sexual behavior could be changed. By re-establishing a classic gay psycho-social sexual script (Nungesser 1983) in line with "pornographic" gay erotica, the communal well-being would somehow be ensured. When pressed, this maladaptive behavior was defined as compulsive because it was believed to stem from such mental states as loneliness or depression, something which impersonal sex would miraculously alleviate.

For GMHC, both the problem and the solution to the sexual transmission of AIDS were individual, subjective, and mechanistic. Thus, there would be no determination of the social fallout and long-term implications (Gagnon 1989) of encouraging impersonal (but safer) sexual encounters for the sake of private pleasure and gain, even when the community interest was generally not fully served, in either good or bad times, by such instrumental activities. However, the program's rationale would be politically acceptable, fundable, and expedient because it dealt with individuals, who were assumed to be responsible, independent, and autonomous actors and whose behavior had no social connections or consequences.

Unwittingly, GMHC's program fitted the political economy of government policymakers who generally prefer to "blame the victim." A psychologically oriented program would also provide easily measurable results while supporting and maintaining the prevailing ideology that pathology, even in a collectively destructive illness like AIDS, primarily resides or emanates in individuals and is not the result of social arrangements. It stands to reason, then, that since GMHC's educational staff was of the Stonewall generation and understood gayness as an issue of personal sexual freedom, that there would be no interest in redefining sexuality and safer-sex in terms of collective needs, that is, as a communal obligation coming from pride, self-acceptance, and collective attachments.

The 800 Men Project further assumed that male sexual behavior is a specialized and independent activity devoid of feelings, contexts, emotions, communal attachments *and* consequences. It supposed a universal type of gay sexuality (Bell and Weinberg 1987), disregarding an individual's social class, education, religious beliefs, and ethnic background. The program's advertising flier depicted two suggestive "butch" gay men. The bottom torso was shown complete with "enviable" penises. This masculine sexual icon, appealing mostly to the gay clone, assumedly represented a normative view of "hot" gay erotica. It ignored the occasional homosexual actor and whole clusters of other types of gays who were, likewise, at risk of both alienating relations and/or AIDS by having unhealthy or unsafe sex. Gay life without the presence of traditional and popular homoerotic interactions (Rechy 1977) was verboten as either an idea or objective at the agency or on the community level. The study again affirmed the idea that gays were not only uniformly homosexual, but uniformly narcissistic. Such views, moreover, leave unchallenged not only sexism and male socialization into instrumentality, but the repression and fear of the overt and affectionate expression of love, desire, and feelings. The joy and pleasure of responsible and authentic self-discovery (Vollmer 1986) is ignored as a goal in safer-sex education.

Given American squeamishness about unorthodox sexual activity and the insistence on containing gay male sexuality (Mass 1981), GMHC hoped to teach gay men how to romanticize condom use, masturbation, and other external and infectiously neutral sexual activities as a solution to unsafe compulsivity. More practically, it encouraged "liberated" gay men to eroticize what would generally be considered tedious or annoying activities like masturbating on a partner's back or chest, sharing an erotic shower or even 'humping' the backs of knee-caps!

A SOCIOLOGICAL REJOINDER

Not only is GMHC's approach depoliticizing, but it leaves instrumental and depersonalized sexual behavior unattended as both a social issue and determinant in AIDS fulmination. Because it did not foster social change by reordering and personalizing relationships within the community (Kruijer 1987), the logic of The 800 Men Project fitted an unliberated understanding of both homosexuality and the politicization process. In fact, if AIDS were not sexually transmitted, patriarchal gay sexual activity would not ever have been considered problematic either for individuals or the community's integration. Former director of the National Lesbian and Gay Task Force, Rosemary Kuropat (1989, p. 17) writes:

> Indeed, the gay movement has rarely been concerned with issues larger than the right (and the means and venues) of gay men to engage in the sex act. An exclusionary AIDS politics simply continues this sex-centricity; never in the twenty years since Stonewall has any force so completely intruded upon that right as has HIV.

Although the texture of human relationships is always affected negatively by impersonality, in terms of AIDS, lodging this behavior in compulsivity and, then, recelebrating it in The 800 Men Project delays the politicization of the community, leaving the structural sources of "maladaptive" sexual behavior unencumbered. If safer-sex education is always political, then it at least needs to be applied consciously in a way that neutralizes homophobia. The 800 Men Project, however, offers an individual adaptation to a collective, communal, and institutional problem. This is dysfunctional because in any social problem, the solution lies in the political process through the reordering of priorities, the redistribution of power, and the reallocation of resources. Essentially, any movement for self preservation that hopes to succeed must make the construction of a collective identity one of its most central tasks (Gamson 1991). As in a holocaust, the community, not just individual actors, is at risk of annihilation (Denneny 1990).

GMHC's solution to maladaptive behavior not only failed to address homophobia, but neglected to identify the way the subjective ideologies and homosexual experiences of its own staff colored the proposal's logic, objectives, and methodologies. GMHC's definition of the problem was value-laden and because it reflected government prejudices about homosexuals actually revealed homophobic conceptions of gay life. Why else accentuate changing individual genital activity as the solution to the institutionally sustained problem of collective alienation and, now, annihilation? This approach shows disregard for the common good and encourages disassociation from the community as a "sacred" source of identity and well-being (Abalos 1986). If the fulmination of AIDS has social consequences, then its containment must be on the structural (political) level by "healing" homophobia personally through the communalization process (Kayal 1990b).

Like any confined people who become what is expected and defined for them by powerful institutions, many gays behave maladaptively. Because of AIDS-induced despair and guilt, this tendency is now exacerbated. The mixing of morals with medicine stigmatized already-tarnished others, depriving them of access to themselves and the community as life-giving, creative sources (Kayal 1985). Gay male sexual activity becomes harmful under such circumstances because psychic and social fragmentation increases by separating the inner self from the community as a legitimate, valued, and authentic 'sacred' source. When there are moralistic pressures to conform to a patriarchal social order, detachment from one's community becomes more likely. In a crisis like AIDS, this is suicidal because having unsafe-sex is directed at the community as a negative source and burdensome entity. This is why it is dangerous and why it needs to be "healed." Unsafe sex is an illness of spirit and soul. It reflects a fractured identity and existence.

Catholic theologian Mary Hunt (1987) attributes this situation to an inhumane "pornographic theology" which denies spontaneity and emotion in relationships and subjugates all sexual activity to reproduction as a norm. Such a corporate, "stateside" theology is inherently homophobic and destructive of mental health.

It leads to exclusion from the national society on moral grounds (Bellah et al. 1985). As a result, many gays take their anger and frustrations out on themselves, that is, on one another. Responsible sexual activity is less likely because their homosexuality is considered problem causing and troublesome.

Being defined as deviant and sinful by powerful religious institutions (Gordon 1986; Hunt 1987) fragments the gay psyche and creates cleavages between the self and the community as its natural extension. When guilt, sex, stigma, fear, and "the god" of orthodox religion meet, the stage is set for the development of maladaptive behavior or an unhealed (self-accepting) psychology. Much of gay sexual behavior immediately before the onslaught of AIDS reflected negative and institutionalized religious images and social expectations (Kayal 1992).

Even now, homosexual encounters often mirror masculine sex roles generally. They frequently emphasize sexual experience as an end in itself, if not the means to a life-long "lover" (Altman 1986, pp. 140-171; Holleran 1988). Understandably, because it was at the time a long-sought-after, life-giving celebration of freedom, it was impossible to imagine that "hot" sex, when impersonal, might be damaging to communal and psychic health, even if done safely. As psychotherapist W. Wedin (1984b) has indicated, internalized homophobia is often expressed as a desire for anonymous sex, the fulfillment of which is directly related to the spread of AIDS.

In any case, sex for its own sake cannot be the basis for either AIDS prevention, group solidarity, or politicization. When mutuality, concern, and compassion are missing from human relationships, the fabric and basis of community are damaged, the politicization process is undermined, and social or institutional change retarded. Impersonal sex is also problematic psychologically because it is instrumental and destroys linkages between partners by not allowing for personal recognition and acceptance; it leaves persons unknown to one another. Impersonal sex fails to recognize the connection between personal relations and communal well-being. On the other hand, personalizing sexual relations will make both impersonal multiple partnering and unsafe sexual practices less likely. While generally true, this assertion is even more significant now because of how discrimination and homophobia intersect with AIDS causality and prevention, thus increasing social isolation and detestable "otherness" (Johnston 1987).

Maladaptive sexual behavior, especially during AIDS, is a response to this exclusion and marginalization. It is the result of the broader, institutional restrictions on holistic relations among men and between men and women. Yet social order "moralists" early on seized the opportunity to blame AIDS on homosexuality rather than even a biological pathogen, never mind social discrimination and prejudice (Martin and Vance 1984). As theories of sperm overload, promiscuity, antibiotic overuse for STDs, excessive recreational drug-use, tears, kissing, intimacy, stroking, and eventually socializing all became suspect, it became obvious that gay expressiveness, if not community, was being attacked and undermined and not the biological causes of AIDS per se. Patton (1985) suggests that the containment of gays, not the prevention of HIV infection became the primary theme in the federal AIDS program.

In effect, safer-sex advocates at GMHC were operating within what sociologists call a social-order model of society (Horton 1966). By devising solutions that promoted safer sexual practices (in terms of AIDS transmission) but which left alienated (instrumental) relations untouched, gay sexual activity would remain shaped by the heterosexist social order, thus reaffirming and reducing gay life and community to sexual activity. There was no acknowledgment that sexual behavior and social life were connected.

Given the political economy of AIDS education in general, GMHC's program was derived from practical necessity, not experience or informed thought. It was fundable and manageable and would appeal to gay activists who were demanding that something be done quickly and cheaply, since no cure was in sight (Barton 1986). If low self-esteem, marginalization, fear, and guilt were also considered as problems, then more confrontational strategies (like those of the AIDS Coalition To Unleash Power) would have to be devised, even though they would not attract grant money or be easily crafted. Yet, to believe that educational programs, including videos and simulation games, could alone resolve this problem was highly naive.

Labelling any sexual behavior as compulsive when it is a response to sexist social conditions actually increases guilt and helplessness and again blames the victim. Given the collective nature of AIDS, it is not appropriate or useful to define people as incurable nymphomaniacs. Doing so assumes that sexually active gays, like "bad girls," are particularly promiscuous and ipso facto degenerate if they sexually engage multiple partners, rather than if they primarily or additionally engage them impersonally, or unsafely.

From a sociological perspective, "compulsive sex" has not been clearly and objectively operationalized except in terms of frequency and numbers of partners. Yet these sexually active individuals are defined as notably depressed, anxious, perhaps even homophobic, and these states of mind are seen as the causative agents rather than products of marginalization and oppression. As a concept, compulsive sex offers neither an explanation or analysis of maladaptive behavior. It is not an empirically verifiable fact but is only an interpretation of behavior, derived from assessments of distraught homosexuals in therapy. It is often applied to homosexual actors who now decide that they are engaging in dangerous, unhealthy sexual activity (Wedin 1984c).

Even if these clinical impressions are valid, sociologically these troubles are the product of what Adam (1978) identifies as the internalized expectations normally associated with inferior status, not compulsive personalities. A patriarchal social order makes an integrated and connected gay life impossible.

It not only forces gay people into exaggerated male roles (and their opposites) but turns victory in competitive sexual activity, performance, and the pursuit of pleasure into primary goals. In this context, maladaptive sexual behavior, rather than being a response to depression, anxiety, and loneliness, is a learned behavior and is the result of accepting one's own subordination and inferiority as part of the natural order of things. Compulsive sex, if it exists, is actually an epiphenomenon, a secondary function of the way maleness is defined in our society. It is the logical product of sexist social arrangements.

Rather than challenge the patriarchal basis of gay male culture and values directly, or endorse abstinence, which would have been tantamount to sociopolitical and communal disintegration, GMHC's educational efforts concentrated on controlling specific transmission modes, as if they were only psychologically determined. In The 800 Men Project, the rationale of individual compulsive sexuality as causative was accepted, though without an appreciation of both the political (structural) and affective (relational) contexts surrounding and supporting such behavior.

In reality sexual behavior, its style, expression, and meaning are intimately tied to social conditions, either in structural terms (the sociopolitical determinants and definition of homosexual behavior in a society) or symbolically (the meaning of sex to the individual actors themselves). It would be unproductive AIDS prevention programming, therefore, not to recognize that in American society, gay male sexual behavior cannot be understood outside the intersection of sexism, male eros, homophobia, and minority status (Kayal and San Giovanni 1984).

As an illness, the specific pathogenic cause of AIDS or its biological mode of transmission are one thing and the conditions and behaviors which allow it to spread and take hold, another. Since AIDS universally is a disease of the disenfranchised, as such, it is rooted in discriminatory social arrangements. In this sense, AIDS has many causes and psychosocial characteristics, not the least of which is sexism, socioeconomic oppression, psychic brokenness, and spiritual despair which, at the very least, incubate and spread HIV (Fortunato 1987). These realities weigh heavily on gays and lesbians and are significant because "the reification of gender and sexual norms, and the stigmatization of difference," as Irvine (1990, pp. 20-21) notes, "are serious endeavors that maintain a social hierarchy of power" over both gay men's and women's lives in general.

In patriarchal culture, the binary opposition of male and female forms the basis of the central organizing hierarchy. Phallocentrism enforces the notion of woman as deficient because of her lack of a penis. Similarly sexual differences like homosexuality, transsexualism, or transvestism are considered deviations that pose a threat to the heterosexual imperative.

The 800 Men Project ignored the fact that sexual behavior becomes maladaptive (and viewed as deviant) when individual sexuality develops or is expressed within an insistent heterosexist and reproductive social order which controls the production of culture and the images a society holds of what is bad, good, normative, and deviant. Rather than encourage healthier social and interpersonal behavior through cementing psychic and social connections, the project required participants to view pictures showing the ugly consequences of infection and illness. The program relied on fear of exposure to the virus as a motivation for changing behavior. Instead of increasing self-esteem, which comes through the establishment of connections to a community that is seen as a concomitant part of the personal self, GMHC attempted to manipulate homoeroticism.[6]

Such psychological prevention programs, however, are designed to make it safe to go on doing what was done before, reinforcing fragmented social relations. In this sense, they are not apolitical. By turning nontransformative and unsafe sex into alienating safer sex and by not acknowledging the false consciousness in gay consciousness, The 800 Men Project actually depoliticized. All GMHC could attempt was "instant community" through reinforced, if not contrived, encouragement and support. GMHC did not try to emphasize making sex safer by putting it into the context of concern and identification with "the other," the disenfranchised and stigmatized gay neighbor. There is, a real difference, nonetheless, between reinforcement in an associational setting and a community wherein common identities, goals, attachments, and relationships are established and valued.

Putting aside the deeper question of prioritizing community concerns instead of individual needs, there are many reasons besides mental illness for being sexually active with many partners which the project ignored, not the least of which are gay male socialization and the natural, erotic satisfaction, enjoyment, and spontaneity of male-to-male sex (Rowland 1986). Age and how long a person has been sexually active, may also explain why some people have anonymous sex with multiple partners. The project also failed to identify that engaging in unsafe sex is a function of perceived risk, which is itself related to both values (or worldview) and the lack of social networks, that is, friends who define reality in a similar way and who may *not* be changing their own behavior or have no personal contact with people who have AIDS.

GMHC's beliefs not withstanding, there are a whole range of intersecting psychosocial variables that affect AIDS transmission (Ceballos-Capitaine et al 1990). For some, AIDS becomes a way out of having to live in a homophobic and hostile world (Martin and Vance 1984). Clearly, AIDS fulmination is facilitated by the intersection of the HIV pathogen with specifically oppressive and discriminatory social environments. Maladaptive behavior (as impersonal multiple partnering or unsafe sexual practices) and AIDS transmission are more likely to occur when the availability of social and sexual options is limited.

The psychoneuroimmunologic dimension of both AIDS transmission and compulsive sexual behavior would be considerably amplified if these factors were taken into consideration (Cohen and Weisman 1986).

SELF- AND COMMUNITY-ACCEPTANCE AND AIDS PREVENTION

Successful and effective AIDS prevention programs require strategies which join individual and collective interests in the "service of transformation" (Halpern 1969), that is, reestablish awareness of the links between overall individual well-being and social structure. Safer-sex education needs to empower the community to take control of its life because it sees itself collectively as an embodiment of something good and sacred; social relationships that empower, embody values of participation and community in their concrete practice (Gamson 1991).

Politicization occurs when gays see the PWA as an extension of themselves and members of the community, with whom their future interests are positively tied (Kayal 1990b). Deepening connections between gays reflect self-acceptance, trust, and familiarity (Singer, Castillo, Davison, and Flores 1990, p. 207). Together, these affect relationships, making safer sex a commitment to the community's longevity. Undoubtedly, however, fostering personal attachment to the collective well-being by putting sexual activity in the context of mutual concern would be too radical to be funded, if it were considered at all. However, if the affective and rational are not successfully integrated together, and both with sexuality and feelings, changes in behavior generally do not last. Emotions are as important as knowledge in determining responsible behavior. As with Latinos, putting on a condom has to become a sign of "respeto." not a sign of mistrust (Carrillo 1988, pp. 12-13). It represents a shift in both feelings and consciousness.

The issue is not whether or not The 800 Men Project was successful for some individuals because it most certainly appeared to be, if not in the long term, then at least temporarily (Gay Men's Health Crisis 1987). Rather, it is its effects on community building and empowerment which are important sociologically because without communalization, the problem cannot be resolved. The question is, then, not whether safer-sex practices can be taught and sustained through individual psychological reconditioning, but whether a social problem like AIDS and its fulmination can be resolved without addressing the deeper structural issues of disempowerment, homophobia, guilt, low self-esteem, and communal rejection. All these fuel maladaptive sexual and social behavior.

While it might be that people are having unsafe sex because they do not know how to behave any other way or because they cannot imagine safer sex to be enjoyable, it is more likely that such activity now occurs among depoliticized and isolated individuals. Undoubtedly, most participants in The 800 Men Project already knew about safer-sex guidelines since they are so widely circulated. It is even possible that some needed more encouragement and peer support, in addition to more information on how to act safely. The emphasis on technical training, nevertheless, only hopefully answers the question of why rational, well-informed, and sexually experienced adults still put themselves and others at risk.[7]

If maladaptive behavior is defined as homophobic activity (rather than a technique failure), then it is a rejection of a collective life, a denial of and isolation from community. Its internalization among gays can only be ended, therefore, by attaching the individual interest to the communal need in a way which restores gays to autonomous jurisdiction over social and political forces affecting community life (Kayal 1991). Tilly (1978, p. 69) defines empowerment as "the process by which a group goes from being a passive collection of individuals to an active participant in public life."

From the perspective of community, what really matters is the quality of gay relations, not the quantity. Without a context, safer-sex techniques are counterproductive. By themselves, they ignore the effects of depersonalized relations on both individual mental health and the communalization process. Likewise, unsafe and impersonal sexual activities are maladaptive by reinforcing self-rejection and communal alienation. It is self-defeating, then, to ignore the sociological factors which make sexual activity an erotic, satisfying, and meaningful social event. What needs to be alleviated in safer-sex education is guilt, internalized homophobia, and low self-esteem. These are all done through identification with a community as a life-giving source. Sexual activities and liaisons that spring from alienated sources are always dysfunctional to personal and social integration. Homophobic sex not only reflects psychic fragmentation but destroys communal integrity, actually leaving gays vulnerable to exploitation.

Alone, emphasizing making sex safer (like merely encouraging the use of clean works among drug users) serves the interests of the political majority. It leaves the social forces shaping dysfunctional behavior blameless in the production of personal problems. Basically, choosing multiple and anonymous sex partners is a function of self-image and reflects powerlessness and fatalism. This is be true for everybody, heterosexual and homosexual alike. As William Shattls, a psychotherapist with a large gay and AIDS practice, notes (Rabinowitz 1990, p. 107), "sex is tied up with identity. To give it up is narcissistic injury." He notes, however, that by choosing to do what feelings dictate over what you know is good for you "ends up causing the torments of hell."

According to *The Wellness Letter* of the University of California at Berkeley (1989, p. 3), more than anything else, "optimism and a sense of control over life's events seem to contribute to health, well-being, and longevity." This is precisely what identification and participation in the life of a community achieves and, in AIDS, it means to voluntarily witness the needs of PWAs. To bear witness in this context means being willing to take on the suffering of others as if it were one's own, but in a way that brings the carepartner and the AIDS sufferer into deep conversation with themselves about their own value or sacredness as human beings.

In a 1986 random survey of 300 GMHC volunteers conducted by this writer to determine motivations for volunteering in AIDS, nearly 23 percent of the respondents strongly agreed that they volunteered at the agency to change their feeling of impotence regarding AIDS and 29 percent agreed this was true for them as well. Nearly 64 percent agreed (and 11.4 percent strongly agreed) that their work "on behalf of PWAs" had increased their "sense of self-worth." In effect, they claimed they became empowered because they were doing something for others. When asked to rank which activities have influenced changes in their sexual activity, nearly 18 percent of the survey respondents said that joining GMHC itself was what most influenced their behavior and 43 percent claimed that it was somewhat influential. However, 29 percent indicated that working with PWAs (seeing the human face of AIDS) was most influential and 33 percent said doing so was somewhat influential in changing their behavior. Nearly 36 percent said that their sense of community pride and responsibility somewhat influenced their behavior, as did 37 percent who said supportive friendship networks helped. But only 11 percent of those volunteers who participated said that The 800 Men Project was most influential. And 20 percent signified that it was somewhat influential.

The largest number of volunteer respondents (60 %), however, indicated that their own instinct for self preservation influenced them the most and 34 percent agreed that volunteering had helped them change their sexual behavior for the better. The same proportion of respondents who were identified as HEALED (self-accepting) and GAYPOLS (gay politicos) also indicated that self-preservation was their major motivation for practicing safe sex. Likewise, those identified as high in community pride (COMPRIDE) indicated that their sense of community responsibility greatly influenced their practice of safer-sex and that The 800 Men Project was the least influential.[8] Given how the personal and collective interests are joined in AIDS, these findings actually support each other since the GAYPOLS, COMPRIDES and HEALED were basically the same individuals.[9]

There is also evidence that people with strong social ties, particularly those that involve work for and with other people in a community, tend to be healthier than those who live in isolation. Apparently, when voluntary helpers or carepartners sense their beneficial effects on others, their health is generally enhanced because feelings of helplessness and depression are diminished, replaced by a sense of self-worth, satisfaction, even exhilaration (Snyder and Omoto 1992). However, it is not a healthy situation when the collective identity becomes suddenly synonymous with illness and death. Trust, the basis of relationships that have feelings attached to them, is violated and the experience of and desire for community becomes suspect. "In AIDS," writes Bayer (1989, p. 79), "the most intimate dimensions of human existence, often the sources of our deepest pleasure, have been welded to the threat of lethal disease."

The solution to maladaptive behavior in general lies for gays, then, in the canceling of shame and fear about being homosexual as reflected in living in a "claimed community," identifying with the problems and goals of the larger gay collectivity, and affirming personhood by bearing witness to others even more disadvantaged. The social fabric, validity, and vitality of the gay community cannot be restored as a sacred source of identity through learning only safer sexual techniques which counter sexual compulsiveness as a psychological deficiency. It requires a fundamental reordering of relationships between the personal self and the community based on mutual acceptance.

CONCLUSION

It is homophobia, rather than sexual compulsiveness, which prevents people from being sexually responsible and discovering their own inner "sacred sources" by identifying with the collectivity that their interests (problems) are connected with. Homophobia, therefore, makes unsafe sexual behavior an antigay, antihuman act, not just an individual pathology. According to Shattls (Rabinowitz 1990, p. 104):

> You're talking about a victim here—about men who are the products of cultural values that say it is not okay to be a homosexual. This is a homophobic culture. It's not surprising when someone who's grown up learning to hide and despise his sexual feelings goes out and behaves self-destructively.

Because it is the gay community, as well as individual homosexuals, that suffers in and from AIDS, the disease is very much a gay man's crisis, if not just physically, then certainly socially and spiritually (Gordon 1988). Because of its collective nature, it requires a transformation in intrapsychic and social linkages. "More precisely," notes Denneny (1990, p. 16), "an epidemic is the occurrence of death as a social event." When this happens, "both the individual and the community are threatened with irreparable loss." To save the community's integrity, personal identity and interpersonal relations need to be politicized and celebrated. Because it must deinstitutionalize homophobia, AIDS prevention means political action by the community for the community, and it is this point which AIDS prevention education often ignores.

Putting sexual relations into the relational context of community creates a collective consciousness, a communal sense of responsibility. When affective community is established between and among people, then the shared or common identity is accepted as positive. And when people identify and feel a part of a larger social entity, then they are likely to see their future tied up with that collectivity (Adkins 1986b). In terms of safer-sex, this linkage translates into an emphasis on not infecting another. Engaging in unsafe sex now is essentially an expression of self-hate or internalized homophobia. Not only is it suicidal, but it also contributes to collective disembodiment. The fear among gays of getting AIDS is best directed to the fear of potentially *giving* AIDS. Whether or not one is HIV positive, responsible sexual behavior now means practicing safer-sex in a way which intentionally teaches pride from the space of respect. It reinforces community by being a shared effort—looking out for one another. This is the real difference between mere homosexual activity, even practicing safer-sex, and a healed and complete gay consciousness.

ACKNOWLEDGMENT

The author gratefully acknowledges the editorial contributions of Professor David Abalos and Michele Kayal. An earlier edition of this paper, titled "Healing Maladaptive Sexual Behavior," was read in New York at the 1986 Convention of the Society for the Study of Social Problems.

NOTES

1. Gay people trust GMHC because it is communally generated and controlled, publicly and positively identified with AIDS, and because it corrects disinformation about the disease and its causation. By providing an opportunity for the community to bear witness to itself, it challenges prevailing moralisms and stereotypes about gays. As a result, it offers a safe psychological and sociological haven where gays and PWAs can unconditionally recognize, engage, and accept one another and in the process heal any internalized homophobia among them.

2. This is not to say that gays and others do not need knowledge about safer sex and how to practice it even with lovers and other intimate and personal sexual partners. Rather, it is the assumption that people have unsafe sex because they do not know how not to and that they could only learn new, safer sexual scripts by learning how to eroticize them that is significant, troublesome, and being questioned here.

3. To be sure, there is a complex and long-term relationship between GMHC and different Latino populations in the city. GMHC was first to publish Spanish language literature as well as educational films on AIDS. GMHC also funds Latino AIDS organizations and shares its expertise with them. However, the agency has been less effective in using a Latino frame of reference in its approach to AIDS education/prevention partially because Latin gays respond to two other reference groups besides the gay community—the larger Hispanic community and the predominately white mainstream society. Many Latino AIDS-related problems are also drug-related and not sexual in origin (Morales 1990, p. 214). Much the same is true of women whose concerns about AIDS have generally been ignored (Gillespie 1991). This changed in early 1991, when dozens of women protested GMHC's biases, pointing out that women are the fastest-growing population at risk of infection. They are underplayed at the educational/prevention policy level not so much because their problems are so unique as because their sexuality is often incomprehensible to "masculinist" men and because it does not usually manifest itself in the instrumental or erotic ways that gay men and GMHC staff are accustomed too.

4.   For reasons of identity or personal definitions of sexuality (Morales 1990) and reticence about publicly discussing sexuality (never mind with gay strangers), GMHC's educational approach would also be less appealing or effective for non-gay, at-risk populations (de Carpio 1990). Since little is known about bi- or homosexuality among minorities or the relationship of class oppression and closeted sexual activity to drug use, "a review of available studies," writes Singer, Castillo, Dovison, and Flores (1990, p. 198), "indicates that Latinos are less adequately served than other populations by mainstream AIDS education programs and consequently tend to exhibit a higher prevalence of misconceptions concerning routes of infection and methods of prevention." Unlike gays, whose sex lives have been microscopically investigated in relation to AIDS transmission, there is considerably less interest in the health and welfare of disinherited racial and ethnic minorities. Likewise, the psychology and demographics of GMHC's staff makes them gay-sensitive, limiting their interest and ability to reach out to women and minority communities with enthusiasm, experience, and ability.

5.   The Centers for Disease Control withheld its pledged support for 25 AIDS educational programs designed to use videos illustrating safer-sex techniques (Adkins 1986; Ford 1986) because they described safer homosexual sex. Explicit heterosexual visuals had been used for decades throughout the country but now the federal government did not want to appear as either supporting, condoning, or encouraging what it saw as basically illegal activities. A short time thereafter, conservative senator Jesse Helms was able to end funding for GMHC safer-sex comics, claiming they were obscene.

6.   Oddly, The 800 Men project was characterized by an inordinate concern with privacy and confidentiality, lest the names of participants become publicly known. Fear of being exposed as a gay person, however, does not facilitate healing and does not encourage the atmosphere from which transformation and community affirmation emerges and maladaptive behavior is curtailed.

7.   Technically, safer sex means avoiding sharing body fluids, IV needles, and infected ejaculate internally. Yet, there are both absolutely strict and more relaxed versions of safer sex. They range from abstinence and condom use for oral sex, to no kissing, the avoidance of pre-ejaculate, and coitus interruptus. Early on, some specialists believed multiple exposures to massive amounts of the virus were necessary, while others claimed a one-shot infection is all that is needed. Oral sex, with or without condoms, is underplayed as a mode of transmission and anal sex, for the passive partner, is universally condemned. Use of latex condoms are generally seen as effective inhibitors of transmission.

8.   In a comparable study of AIDS volunteers in Minnesota, psychologists Snyder and Omoto (1992) write that they have every reason to expect that "as a result of working in AIDS organizations, volunteers should develop more favorable attitudes towards PWAs, have decreased fear and increased knowledge about AIDS, become more likely to practice safer-sex behaviors, and be more likely to engage in AIDS-related activism (e.g., monetary donations, lobbying)."

9.   In organizing the results of a 14-page questionnaire measuring attitudes, knowledge about AIDS, homophobia, nurturing skills, community involvement, and motivations for volunteering, respondents fell into general, but not mutually exclusive, categories. People who were HEALED did not see AIDS as a punishment from God, embraced their homosexuality, identified with the community, and were not afraid of the stigma attached to AIDSWORK. Those who were COMPRIDE volunteered because they wanted to identify with the community and its problems and were involved with community institutions. The GAYPOLS were generally gay activists, especially in AIDS. When cross-tabulated, the same respondents emerged in each category.

REFERENCES

Abalos, D. 1986. *Latinos in the United States.* Notre Dame: University of Notre Dame Press.
Adam, B. 1978. *The Survival of Domination.* New York: Elsevier.

Adkins, B. 1986a. "GMHC Accepts Grant from CDC for Sex Education Research." *The New York Native.* 147(February 10-16): 8.

————. 1986b. "Liquor May be Quicker, But Pride is Just Dandy." *The New York Native.* 161(May 19): 18.

Altman, D. 1982. *The Homosexualization of America.* New York: St. Martins Press.

————. 1986. *AIDS in the Mind of America.* New York: Doubleday.

Barnett, A. 1986. "Saving Sex." *The New York Native.* 167(May 19): 17.

Barton, K.D. 1986. "The Phallacy of Waiting for a Cure for AIDS." *The New York Native.* 146(February 3-9): 25-26.

Bell, A. and M. Weinberg. 1978. *Homosexualities: A Study of Diversity Among Men and Women.* New York: Simon and Schuster.

Bellah, R. 1985. *Habits of the Heart.* Berkeley, CA: University of California.

Brandt, A.M. 1985. *No Magic Bullet: A Social History of Venereal Disease.* New York: Oxford University Press.

Carrillo, E. 1988. "AIDS and the Latino Community." *Centro Bulletin* 3: 7-14.

Ceballos-Capitaine, A., J. Szapocznik, N. Blaney et al. 1990. "Ethnicity, Emotional Distress, Stress-Related Disruption, and Coping Among HIV Seropositive Gay Males." *Hispanic Journal of Behavioral Science* 12(2, May): 135-152.

Cohen, M.A. and H.W. Weisman. 1986. "A Biopsychosocial Approach to AIDS." *Psychosomatics* 27(4, April): 245-249.

de Carpio, A.B. and F. Carpio-Cedrano, and L. Anderson. 1990. "Hispanic Families Learning and Teching About AIDS: A Participatory Approach at the Community Level." *Hispanic Journal of Behavioral Sciences* 12(2, May): 165-176.

Denneny, M. 1990. "A Quilt of Many Colors: AIDS Writing and the Creation of Culture." *Christopher Street* 12(9, 141): 15-21.

Ford, D. 1986. "CDC Rejects Safe-Sex Film Hands Down." *The New York Native.* 146(February 3-9): 13.

Fortunato, J.E. 1983. *Embracing the Exile.* New York: Seabury Press.

————. 1987. *AIDS: The Spiritual Dilemma.* New York: Harper & Row.

Friedman, S. and J.L. Sotheran, L. Abdul-Quader, et al. 1987. "The AIDS Epidemic Among Blacks and Hispanics. *The Millbank Quarterly* 65 (Supplement 2): 455-499.

Fumento, M. 1989. *The Myth of Heterosexual AIDS.* New York: Basic Books.

Gagnon, J. 1990. "Disease and Desire." *Daedalus* 118(2, Spring): 47-78.

Galliher, J.F., and C. Tyree. 1985. "Edwin Sutherland's Research on the Origins of Sexual Psychopath Laws: An Early Case Study of the Medicalization of Deviance." *Social Problems* 33(2, December): 100-113.

Gamson, W. 1991. "Commitment and Agency in Social Movements." *Sociological Forum* 6(1): 27-50.

Gay Men's Health Crisis. 1987. *Report: "The 800 Men Project." New York: GMHC*

————. 1989. *The Annual Report.* New York: GMHC.

Gillespie, M.A. 1991. "HIV: The Global Crisis." *Ms. Magazine* 1(4, January-February): 17-23

Greenberg, D. 1988. *The Construction of Homosexuality.* Chicago: The University of Chicago Press.

Gordon, K., ed. 1986. *Homosexuality and Social Justice.* San Francisco, CA: The Consultation.

————. 1988. "Can There Be Faith and Theology After AIDS?" Paper presented in the James Memorial Chapel, Union Theological Seminary, April 16.

————. 1989. "The Sexual Bankruptcy of the Christian Tradition: A Perspective of Fundamental Trust." Pp. 169-213 in *AIDS Issues: Confronting the Challenge,* edited by D.G. Hallman. New York: Pilgrim Press.

Halpern, M. 1969. "A Redefinition of the Revolutionary Situation. *Journal of International Affairs* XXIII(1): 54-75.

Hammonds, E. 1987. "Race, Sex, AIDS: The Construction of Other." *Radical America* 20(6): 28-36.
Holleran, A. 1988. *Ground Zero*. New York: New American Library.
Horton, J. 1966. "Order and Conflict Theories of Social Problems As Competing Ideologies." *American Journal of Sociology* 71(May): 701-713.
Hunt, M. 1987. "Theological Pornography: From Corporate to Communal Ethics." Paper presented at a seminar of The Consultation, Union Theological Seminary.
Irvine, J. 1990. *Disorders of Desire: Sex and Gender in American Sexology*. Philadelphia, PA: Temple University.Press.
Johnston, G. 1979. *Which Way Out of the Men's Room?* Cranberry, NJ: A.S. Barnes & Co.
Johnston,R. Jr., 1987. "AIDS and 'Otherness.'" Pp. 77-83 in *AIDS: Public Policy Dimensions,* edited by J. Griggs. New York: United Hospital Fund.
Kayal, P. 1985. "Morals, Medicine and the AIDS Epidemic." *Journal of Religion and Health* 24(3): 218-238.
――――― 1990a. "American Volunteer Ideology, AIDS and the Community." Paper presented at the Convention of the Eastern Sociological Society, Boston, March 24.
――――― 1990b. "Healing Brokenness: Gay Volunteerism in AIDS," *Humanity and Society* 14(3, August): 280-296.
――――― 1991. "Gay/AIDS Volunteerism as Political Activity." *The Nonprofit and Voluntlary Sector Quarterly* 20(3): 289-312.
――――― 1992. "Healing Homophobia: 'the Sacred' in AIDS Volunteerism." *Journal of Religion and Health* 31(2): 113-128.
Kayal, P. and L. San Giovanni. 1984. "Objectivity in the Sociology of Sexuality: Sexism and Homophobia." *Free Inquiry into Creative Sociology* 12(2, November): 161-166.
Kobasa, S.C. 1990. "AIDS and Volunteer Associations: Perspectives on Social and Individual Change." *Millbank Quarterly* 68(Supplement 2): 280-294.
Kruijer, G. 1987. *Development Through Liberation*. Atlantic Highlands, NJ: Humanities Press.
Kuropat, R. 1989. "Response to Darrel Yates Rist." *Christopher Street* 11(11, 132): 17-18.
Levine, M. 1979. "Gay Ghetto." Pp. 182-204 in Gay Men, edited by M. Levine. New York: Harper & Row.
Marin, B.V., G.Marin, and R. Juarez. 1990. "Differences Between Hispanics and Non-Hispanics in Willingness to Provide AIDS Prevention Advice." *Hispanic Journal of Behavioral Sciences* 12(2, May): 153-164.
Martin, J.L. and C.S. Vance. 1984. "Behavioral and Psychosocial Factors in AIDS: Methodological and Substantive Issues." *The American Psychologist* 39(11): 1-6.
Mass, L. 1981. "A Nation of Sexual Stutterers: A Conversation with Mary Calderone." *Christopher Street* (September/October): 31-35.
Mills, C. W. 1959. *The Sociological Imagination*. New York: Oxford.
Morales, E.S. 1990. "HIV Infection and Hispanic Gay and Bisexual Men." *Hispanic Journal of Behavioral Sciences* 12(2, May): 212-223.
Nungesser, L.G. 1983. *Homosexual Acts, Actors, and Identities*. New York: Praeger.
Palmer, J. L. and I. V. Sawhill, eds. 1984. *The Reagan Record*. Cambridge, MA: Ballinger Press.
Patton, C. 1985. *Sex and Germs*. Boston, MA: South End Press.
Poirier, R. 1988. "AIDS and the Traditions of Homophobia." *Social Research* 55(August): 461-476.
Quadland, M. 1983. "Overcoming Sexual Compulsion." *The New York Native* 76(November 7-20): 25-26.
Rabinowitz, D. 1990. "The Secret Sharer: A Women Confronts her Homosexual Husband's Death from AIDS." *New York Magazine* 23(8, February 26): 102-112.
Rechy, J. 1977. *The Sexual Outlaw*. New York: Grove Press.

Rothschild-Whitt, J. 1979. "The Collectivistic Organization: An Alternative to Rational Bureaucratic Models." *American Sociological Review* 44(4): 519-523.

Rowland, G. 1986. "Reinventing the Sex Maniac." *The Advocate.* (January 21):, 43-49.

See, B. 1987. "Treasurer's Report." *GMHC Volunteer Newsletter* 4(4, July/August): 2.

Shilts, R. 1987. *And the Band Played On.* New York: St. Martin's Press.

Singer, M., Z. Castillo, L. Davison, and C. Flores. 1990. "Owning AIDS: Latino Organizations and The AIDS Epidemic." *Hispanic Journal of Behavioral Sciences* 12(2, May): 196-211.

Snyder, M. and A.M. Omoto. 1992. "Who Helps and Why?: The Psychology of AIDS Volunteerism." Pp. 219-239 in *Helping and Being Helped: Naturalistic Studies,* edited by S. Oskamp, and S. Spacapan. Newbury Park, CA: Sage.

Tilly, C. 1978. *From Mobilization to Revolution.* Reading, MA: Addison-Wesley.

University of California. 1989. "Help Others, Help Yourself." *The Wellness Letter* (University of California at Berkeley, School of Public Health) 6(2): 3.

Vollmer, T. 1986. "Why Gay Liberation Turned Against Us." *The New York Native* 185 (April 28): 23-25.

Wedin, W. 1984a. "The Sexual Compulsion Movement." *Christopher Street* 8(3, 88) 48-54.

_____ 1984b. "Scxual Healing." *The New York Native* 95(July 30): 26-29.

_____ 1984c. "No Cure for Anonymous Sex." *The New York Native* 87: 21, 36.

Weinberg, G. 1973. *Society and the Healthy Homosexual.* New York: Doubleday.

BIOGRAPHICAL SKETCHES

Peter Aggleton is Director of the Health and Education Research Unit at Goldsmiths' College, University of London. He is actively involved in research in the field of HIV/AIDS health promotion and directs projects funded by the World Health Organization, the Health Education Authority, the Economic and Social Research Council and the AIDS Education and Research Trust (AVERT). Current research interests include the interface between lay and professional knowledge about HIV/AIDS, the effectiveness of interventions to reach non-gay men who have sex with men and the monitoring and evaluation of local HIV/AIDS health promotion. His recent publications include *Deviance* (Tavistock, 1987), *Social Aspects of AIDS* (edited with H. Homans) (Falmer Press, 1988), *Health* (Routledge, 1990), *AIDS: Responses, Interventions and Care* (edited with P. Davies and G. Hart) (Falmer Press, 1991).

Gary L. Albrecht is a Professor in the School of Public Health at the University of Illinois-Chicago. His current work examines how emotions, risks, stigma, and cultural context affect social responses to AIDS. He has worked with the Global Programme on AIDS of the World Health Organization in Geneva, Switzerland, and Project Hope in Washington, D.C., since 1987 on international AIDS studies. His most recent book is *The Disability Business* (Sage, 1992). He was chair of the Medical Sociology section of the American Sociological Association, 1987-1988, and Academic Visitor, Nuffield College, Oxford University, 1992.

Judith K. Barr is Associate Director for Programs at the New York Business Group on Health and Adjunct Associate Professor at the Robert F. Wagner Graduate School of Public Service, New York University. Her recent research concerns working women and stress, employee and employer views about HIV/AIDS in the workplace, eldercare programs in the workplace, and the impact of HIV/AIDS on hospital residency selection. Among her publications are papers in the *Journal of Health and Social Behavior, Social Science and Medicine* and the *Journal of Occupational Medicine*. She received her doctorate from Johns Hopkins University.

Mary Boulton is Senior Lecturer in Sociology as Applied to Medicine at St. Mary's Hospital Medical School, London. Her current research work includes the health beliefs and health behavior of gay men in response to AIDS and the sexual behavior and social experience of bisexual men. She is a consultant to the WHO on bisexuality and HIV transmission. Other research interests include doctor-patient communication and health education in general practice. She is author of *On Being a Mother* (Tavistock, 1983) and *Meetings Between Experts: An Approach to Sharing Ideas in Medical Consultations* (with D. Tuckett, C. Olsen and A. Williams) (Tavistock, 1985).

Robert S. Broadhead is an Associate Professor of Sociology at the University of Connecticut, Storrs. He is working on two books based on the field research: *The Significance of the Gesture: Combating AIDS Among Injection Drug Users* and *FlagShip Down: The Scuttling of a Model AIDS Prevention Project.* An article, "Social Constructions of Bleach in Combating AIDS Among Injection Drug Users," is in the *Journal of Drug Issues* (January 1992).

Stephen Crystal is Associate Research Professor; Director, AIDS Research Group; and Chair, Division on Aging, at the Institute for Health, Health Care Policy, and Aging Research at Rutgers University. His research on formal and informal care provision in AIDS has encompassed a series of surveys of persons with AIDS in San Diego and New Jersey. He was principal investigator of the needs assessment survey of persons with AIDS in New Jersey and is currently principal investigator of a longitudinal study of health care costs and utilization in a cohort of New Jersey PWAs.

Ray Fitzpatrick is University Lecturer in Medical Sociology and a Fellow of Nuffield College, Oxford. His current research work includes the health beliefs and health behavior of gay and bisexual men in response to AIDS and the social and psychological aspects of rheumatoid arthritis. Other research interests include theoretical and methodological aspects of research on patient satisfaction, health status and quality of life. His publications include *The*

Experience of Illness (with J. Hinton, S. Newman, G. Scambler and J. Thompson) (Tavistock, 1985) and articles in a wide range of journals.

Kathryn J. Fox is a Doctoral Candidate in Sociology at the University of California, Berkeley. She is the author of two articles in the *Journal of Contemporary Ethnography:* "Real Punks and Pretenders" (1987) and, with Robert S. Broadhead, "Takin' It to the Streets: AIDS Outreach as Ethnography" (1990). Another article, "The Politics of Prevention: Ethnographers Reach Out to IV Drug Users," is published in *Ethnography Unbound* (edited by Michael Burawoy) (University of California Press, 1991).

Samuel R. Friedman is a Senior Principal Investigator at Narcotic and Drug Research, Inc. He has been involved in AIDS research since 1983, focusing primarily on HIV epidemiology and prevention issues concerning drug injectors, and on racial dynamics that affect the HIV epidemic. He has been a co-chair of the Sociology AIDS Network (1986-89), a member of the steering committee of the International Working Group on Drug Use and AIDS (1986-present), a member of the Board of Directors of the Society for the Study of Social Problems (1980-83), chair of the Labor Studies Division of the SSSP (1977-79), and co-chair of the Marxist Sociology Division of the American Sociological Association (1987-88). He is also a published poet.

Deborah C. Glik is an assistant professor in the School of Public Health, University of California-Los Angeles. Her current research interests include perceptions of risk, child safety, psychosocial factors in the use of alternative and religious healers, international health, and the relationship between social roles and wellness.

Claudine Herzlich is Directeur de Recherches au National Center for Scientific Research (CNRS) and teaches at the Ecole des Hautes Etudes en Sciences Sociales. She is the author of Médecine, Maladie, Société (Mouton-EHESS, 1970) *Health and Illness, A Sociological Analysis* (Academic Press, 1973) *Le sens du mal* (with Marc Augé) (Editions des Archives Contemporaines, 1984) *Illness and Self in Society* (with Janine Pierret) (The Johns Hopkins University Press, 1987), and of many articles. She works in Paris in CERMES (Centre de Recerche Médecine, Maladie et Sciences Sociales), a research centre supported by CNRS and INSERM (National Institute of Health and Medical Research).

Kirby Jackson is an instructor in the Department of Epidemiology and Biostatistics, School of Public Health, University of South Carolina. He has special interests in biostatistical aspects of studies in child safety, perceptions of risk, and adolescent mental health issues.

Professor Philip M. Kayal is a Professor of Sociology at Seton Hall University. Concentrating his studies in the sociology of religion and ethnic/minority relations, he received his Ph.D. from Fordham University in 1970. In 1975, he published *The Syrian-Lebanese in America: A Study of Religion in Assimilation*. In addition to numerous articles on the social experiences of Arab-Americans, he has also published widely in the area of gay studies, and now, AIDS. His emphasis is the mobilization of the gay community through the Gay Men's Health Crisis, Inc., in New York City. A research project assessing the meaning of gay/AIDS volunteerism was begun in 1986 and a book titled *Bearing Witness: The AIDS Volunteer as Political Innovator* is being prepared for publication. Several chapters and summary points have recently been published in journals as diverse as *The Journal of Religion and Health, Humanity and Society,* and *The Nonprofit Sector Quarterly.*

Jennie Jacobs Kronenfeld is a Professor in the School of Health Administration and Policy, Arizona State University. Her current research interests include perceptions of risk, childhood injury, the relationship between social roles and wellness, and health policy studies, especially on the impact of DRG's on health care delivery and access to care issues.

Janine Pierret is Chargé de Recherches au National Center for Scientific Research (CNRS). She serves on the editorial board of Sciences Sociales et Santé. She is co-author of *Illness and Self in Society* (with Claudine Herzlich) (The Johns Hopkins University Press, 1987), and she has written many articles. She works in Paris for CERMES (Centre de Recerche Médecine, Maladie et Sciences Sociales), a research centre supported by CNRS and INSERM (National Institute of Health and Medical Research).

Nina Glick Schiller is Assistant Professor of Anthropology at the University of New Hampshire. She was previously a member of the AIDS Research Group at the Institute for Health, Health Care Policy and Aging Research at Rutgers University, where she was project director for the needs assessment survey of persons with AIDS in New Jersey.

Rose Weitz is Professor of Sociology at Arizona State University, specializing in sociology of health, deviance, and gender. She is the editor of *The Sociology of AIDS: A Set of Syllabi and Related Materials* (American Sociological Association), the author of *Life with AIDS* (Rutgers University Press, 1991), and Chair of the Sociologists' AIDS Network.

Rick Zimmerman is Associate Professor of Sociology at the University of Miami, Coral Gables, Florida. His areas of specialization include medical sociology, methods/statistics, and social psychology. His current research includes a multi-site study of knowledge, attitudinal, belief, and skill predictors of AIDS-related risk behavior among clients of sexually transmitted disease clinics; evaluation of a training program for mental health professionals on HIV/AIDS; evaluation for a psychoeducational program for women who are pregnant or post-partum, HIV+, and have a history of chemical dependency; and a large longitudinal school survey assessing sociocultural precursors of substance use and delinquency among adolescents. Long-term research interests center around models of health promotion and disease prevention. He served as Chair of the Sociologists' AIDS Network, 1990-1991.

Advances in Medical Sociology

Edited by **Gary L. Albrecht,** *School of Public Health, University of Illinois at Chicago*

This series, *Advances in Medical Sociology* is dedicated to publishing innovative current research and cutting edge conceptual papers in the broad ranging arena of the Sociology of Health. The papers in these volumes provide new insights into established research areas and open new topics and problems for investigation. These annual volumes are intended to stimulate further creative research.

Volume 1, 1990, 329 pp.　　　　　　　　　　　　$73.25
ISBN I-55938-092-6

Volume 2, 1991, 322 pp. $73.25
ISBN 1-55938-252-X

Edited by **Gary L. Albrecht and Judith A. Levy,** *School of Public Health, University of Illinois at Chicago*

JAI PRESS INC.

55 Old Post Road - No. 2   P.O. Box 1678
Greenwich, Connecticut 06836-1678
Tel: (203) 661-7602   Fax: (203)661-0792

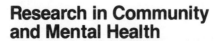

Research in Community and Mental Health

Edited by **James R. Greenley,** *Department of Psychiatry and Sociology, University of Wisconsin* and **Philip J. Leaf,** *School of Epidemiology and Public Health, Yale University*

REVIEWS: ". . . as a whole this is an excellent collection of research articles on several issue important to the field of mental health—mental disorder."

— *Contemporary Sociology*

". . . professionals looking for high quality empirical studies that carry on long standing research traditions will find much value in this collection."

— *Contemporary Psychology*

Volume 6, Mental Disorders in Social Context
1990, 436 pp. $73.25
ISBN 0-89232-726-X

Volume 7, 1992 325 pp. $73.25
ISBN 1-55938-441-7

CONTENTS: PART I. LITERATURE REVIEWS ON SPECIAL ISSUES: HOMELESSNESS AND ETHNICITY. **Mental Illness Among Homeless Adults: A Synthesis of Recent NIMH-Funded Research,** *Richard C. Tessler and Deborah L. Dennis.* **Ethnic Minority Mental Health Service Delivery: A Review of the Literature,** *Harold W. Neighbors.* **PART II. SOCIAL FACTORS AND MENTAL ILLNESS IN COMMUNITY POPULA-TIONS. Somatization and Hypochondraiasis: Sociocultural Factors in Subjective Experience,** *Ronald J. Angel and Ellen L. Idler.* **Cross-Cultural Aspects of Psychotic Symptoms in Puerto Rico,** *Peter J. Guarnaccia, Luz M. Guevara-Ramos, Glorida Gonzales, Glorisa J. Canino, and Hector Bird.* **The Exposure and Vulnerability of Ethnic Minorities to Life Events,** *David T. Takeuchi and Russell K. Adair.* **Gender, Marital Status and Depression,** *Joy Perkins Newmann and Dorothy Watson.* **PART III. CARING FOR PERSONS WITH MENTAL DISORDERS IN THE COMMUNITY. Sheltering the Severely Mentally Ill in the Community: A Sequential Decision Model,** *Gene A. Fisher, Richard C. Tessler, Ronald W. Manderscheid, and Ira B. Sommers.* **Caregiver Network Structure and Access to Informal Support for the Mentally Ill,** *Mark Tausig, David J. O'Brien, and Shubhasree Subedi.* **Illness Theory and Illness Identity: Explaining Compliance Behavior of Epileptic Patients,** *K.V. Kirchgssler.* **Community-Oriented Rehabilita-tion of Mental Patients in West Germany: Case Studies,** *Peter Novak.* **PART IV. ADVANCES IN RESEARCH METHODS. Sources of Attenuation in the Stress-Distress Relationship: An Evaluation of Modest Innovations in the Application of Event Checklists,** *R. Jay Turner and William R. Avison.* **Spurious Associations in Longitudinal Research,** *Bruce G. Link and Patricia E. Shrout.*

Also Available:
Volumes 1-5 (1979-1984) $73.25 each

JAI PRESS INC.

55 Old Post Road - No. 2   P.O. Box 1678
Greenwich, Connecticut 06836-1678
Tel: (203) 661-7602   Fax: (203)661-0792

Research in the Sociology of Health Care

Edited by **Dorothy C. Wertz**, *School of Public Health, Boston University*

Volume 9, 1991, 353 pp. $73.25
ISBN 1-55938-098-5

Also Available:

Volumes 1-8 (1980-1989)
  + Supplement 1 (1981) $73.25 each

Perspectives on Social Problems

Edited by **James A. Holstein** and **Gale Miller**,
Department of Social and Cultural Sciences,
Marquette University

Volume 4, 1992, 299 pp. $73.25
ISBN 1-55938-559-6

Also Available:
Volumes 1-3 (1989-1991) $73.25 each

JAI PRESS INC.

55 Old Post Road - No. 2   P.O. Box 1678
Greenwich, Connecticut 06836-1678
Tel: (203) 661-7602   Fax: (203)661-0792

Current Research on Occupations and Professions

Edited by **Helena Znaniecka Lopata,** *Center for Comparative Study of Social Roles, Loyola University,*

Volume 7, 1992, 252 pp. $73.25
ISBN 1-55938-402-6

Edited by **Gale Miller,** *Marquette University.*

CONTENTS: Introduction. **PART I. PERSPECTIVES ON HUMAN SERVICE OCCUPATIONS AND PROFESSIONS. Human Service Practice as Social Problems Work,** *Gale Miller.* **Producing People: Descriptive Practice in Human Service Work,** *James A. Holstein.* **Influence Work in Human Services Settings: Lessons from the Marketplace,** *Robert Prus.* **PART II. STUDIES OF HUMAN SERVICE PRACTICES.** Professional **Idealizations and Clinical Realities,** *Courtney L. Marlaire.* **Talk-As-Work: The Case of Paramedics for Emergency Field Orders,** *Wayne Martin Mellinger.* **Stretching the Bureaucratic Frame: Careers Interviews in Special Schools,** *David Hughes.* **PART III. STUDIES OF HUMAN SERVICE CAREER CHOICE AND SATISFACTION. Career Change and Identity: Nurse Practitioners' Accounts of Occupational Choice,** *Kathleen Grove.* **Work Autonomy, Organizational Autonomy, and Physicians' Job Satisfaction,** *John C. Lammers.* **Shelter Staff Satisfaction with Services, The Service Network and Their Jobs: The Influence of Disposition and Situation,** *Russell K. Schutt and Mary L. Fennell.* **PART IV. STUDIES OF HUMAN SERVICE PROFESSIONALISM AND PROFESSIONALIZA-TION.** Midwifes in Comparative Perspective: Professionalism in Small Organizations, *Cecelia Benoit.* **Professional Dominance and the Threat of Corporatization,** *Kathleen Montgomery.* **The Deprofessionalization of American Medicine,** *James A. Anderson.*

Also Available:
Volumes 1-6 (1980-1991) $73.25 each

JAI PRESS INC.

55 Old Post Road - No. 2   P.O. Box 1678
Greenwich, Connecticut 06836-1678
Tel: (203) 661-7602   Fax: (203)661-0792